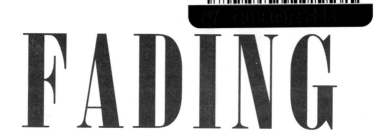

FADING

One family's journey with a woman silenced by

ALZHEIMER'S

Frances A. Kraft

also with

**Preventative, Nutritional & Psychological Help
for the Families and Patients
with Alzheimer's Disease**

Beth M. Ley, Ph.D.
Barry Kraft, D.O.

BL Publications
Detroit Lakes, MN

BL Publications, Detroit Lakes, MN
1-877-BOOKS11/218-826-2519
email: blpub@tekstar.com
Printed in the United States of America
First edition, Jan 2001

Library of Congress Cataloging-in-Publication Data

Kraft, Frances A., 1945-
  Fading: one family's journey with a woman silenced by
Alzheimer's /
Frances A. Kraft, Barry Kraft, Beth M. Ley.-- 1st ed.
      p. cm.
Includes bibliographical references and index.
ISBN 1-890766-14-3 (alk. paper)
1. Reinstein, Maxine Audrey, d. 1984. 2. Alzheimer's
disease--Patients--Biography. 3. Alzheimer's disease--Religious
aspects--Christianity. 4. Alzheimer's disease--Patients--Family
relationships. 5. Christian life. I. Kraft, Barry, 1943- II. Ley,
Beth M., 1964- III. Title.
  RC523.2 .R45 K73 2000
  362.1'96831'0092--dc21
                                              00-010711

Credits:
Cover Design: BL Publications
Typesetting and design work: BL Publications
Proofreading: Debra Brenk, Virginia Simpson-Magruder, and my
daughter Brandy

Special thanks to:
My family: Barry, Max, Brandy and Dirk, without whose unwavering love and support this would've been a *Mission Impossible.*

The Krafts: Anne, George, Michael, Janet and Honey, for your
encouragement.

Madeline Harris, my mentor, who believed in me.

Chuck and Tressa Miville, for your spiritual guidance and fellowship.

Josh Moss, who volunteered hours of his time to help me on the
computer.

Now & Then, who filled my mother's life with music.

Hospice of the Comforter Staff: Ron, Rita, Peggy and Maria, for
your dedication to the highest quality of care for my mother.

Stan, for loving Moose.

Billy's Pizza and Mekong Restaurants, for feeding my mother in
more ways than one.

"THE MOOSE BOOK"

This book is dedicated in loving memory to:

*My mother, Moose. You were a remarkable woman.
I always knew I'd write about you.*

*My father, Max, who taught me to stand up and
be counted.*

*Cheryl Walker, who died at age 48 just 6 months
after my mother. I miss you.*

TABLE OF CONTENTS

My mother, Moose, had been dead three weeks when I checked into the 5-star hotel to read over two hundred letters she had written. It was a date with my past. Her letters chronicled our family events for over thirty years. Once a prolific writer and communicator, she died unable to say more than "lalalala." She was silenced by Alzheimer's.

Five years ago my mother, living in Boca Raton, Florida, began exhibiting bazaar behaviors. We visited her four times that year to assess the problem and come up with a solution.

On our last visit, a startling revelation enabled us to convince Moose that she needed to leave Florida. In four days we had her packed and moved to Colorado.

Considering my mother's age and the dramatic events surrounding her move, she adapted to new surroundings with ease.

We had become part of Moose's delusional system, she called Reuben and told him we had kidnapped her.

Suffering from delusions, Moose tried to run away. We were able to intervene and have her committed to a hospital for diagnosis.

The most appropriate way to handle Moose's affairs, since my brother and I weren't communicating, was to have the state appoint a conservator to handle her finances and hire home health care workers to assist with her daily care.

Chapter VIII: In The Trenches.
Soon, even with all the assistance, Moose couldn't live alone anymore. She needed closer supervision. Being on duty 24/7 required more adjustments.

Chapter IX: Patience Is An Eight Letter Word.
Certain behaviors began to manifest that pushed my buttons. The more I prayed for patience the more behaviors arose that required my patience. At this point I began a journal.

Chapter X: Enter: The Girls.
The more responsibility we took on, the more we recognized we needed help to alleviate some of the pressure. We hired Tammy and Rosie.

Chapter XI: Good Things Happen Too.
At this time our daughter became engaged and we all looked forward to the wedding.

Chapter XII: The Fall.
Unable to monitor my mother's nocturnal habit of wandering, she fell and broke her pelvis. Complications set in and we took my mother home to die.

Chapter XIII:
Chicken Soup –The Ninth Wonder Of The World.
We were told my mother wasn't able to swallow anymore. It was suggested that a feeding tube be inserted in her stomach to sustain her. We rejected any artificial means of keeping her alive and began our chicken soup and love therapy.

Chapter XIV: Welcome To Lalala Land.
One of the by-products of her latest battles to survive was the development of a condition called Echolalia, the constant repetition of a sound.

Chapter XV: Life Goes On.
I found myself enmeshed in wedding plans. As if this weren't enough, we sold our home and moved to a home with easier access for Moose's wheelchair. To assist with Moose's increased care, we had "the girls" move in with us.

This period of preparing for the wedding left me feeling schizophrenic. I was losing my daughter and my mother. In the space of seconds I'd go from feeling elated to overwhelming sadness.

Life was not without giggles. There were many humorous incidents that kept me sane. Moose, for instance, insisted that it was she who was getting married and wanted to buy a wedding gown.

After the wedding we took a trip to visit Moose's sister in Texas and invited her to come live with us.

I've lived long enough to realize that peaceful periods in life are brief. I was still basking in the afterglow of the wedding when we discovered "the girls" were abusing Moose. Action was swift.

We would never have live-in help again. Instead, we hired people for shift work. God sent us Cheryl Walker who entered our lives and took control.

In March Moose died. I was not ready to let go. Barry resuscitated her back and we were all granted a reprieve. God showed great compassion that day.

At the urging of my family, we left Moose in Cheryl's care and took a vacation.

Mother's Day was approaching. I knew it would be our last. I wanted to publicly tell her how much I loved her and not wait until her funeral. I decided to have a living tribute to her. I am forever grateful I did that, because she died a month later.

FOREWORD

Maxine Audrey Reinstein, who was known as "Moose," came into our lives while I was co-pastor with my husband, Charles R. Miville.

We were asked by Dr. Barry Kraft and Fran Kraft if we would consider pastoring church services in their home. It was becoming more difficult for them to attend church as their responsibilities as caregivers for Fran's mother, Moose, in advanced stages of Alzheimer's, increased.

We agreed to conduct a home church for as long as they needed us. It was not difficult to share a small part in Moose's life. We had just completed eleven years as caregivers for my own mother, who had also been a victim to Alzheimer's and had passed away the year before.

Moose was very easy to love. There was a warmth in her smile and wisdom emanated from her eyes. We shared this song called "The Apple Tree." It went like this: "I love you and you love me, we live together in an apple tree." I would make up other words and together Moose and I would sing our song to whomever would listen.

This was a big achievement for Moose to sing "The Apple Tree" song, however simplistic, because of her increased difficulty in speaking. Despite the difficulty she was experiencing, we were establishing a line of communication that comes to those who are making their last journey homeward bound. Yes, there is a language without words that comes to those who are leaving this earth and those who are saying good-bye.

The Krafts called us to their home as Moose

slipped into a coma. That night was lit up with the glory of the Lord as we entered into Moose's bedroom. She was getting ready to continue her journey without us. The Angels were posted by her bedside waiting to usher her into the presence of the Lord. Music filled the air as Frances and I sat quietly soaking in the splendor that was so holy, it just took your breath away.

We will always remember the woman known as Moose. She left her imprints within our hearts. She was such a lady, filled with a spark–fiery, blunt and full of life. She was a masterpiece created by the Lord. It was a privilege to have been part of her final journey.

Dr. Tresa Lena Miville
Pastor Charles R. Miville
House of New Life

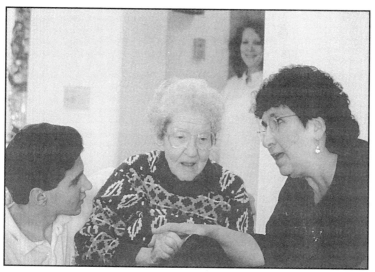

Max and Tresa with Moose.

INTRODUCTION

Have you ever forgotten a word mid-sentence? Have you ever walked into a room and not remembered why you're there? That temporary lapse of memory may have caused you a fleeting feeling of frustration. Imagine if that word you were groping for was erased from your memory forever, replaced with "watchamacallit" or "thingamajig" or your entire day was filled with unfamiliar faces and places. That is the terrifying world of the AD (Alzheimer's Disease) patient. Their life is like a camera lens that keeps getting smaller and darker as their skills diminish.

AD is the fourth leading cause of death in adults. Today there are 4 million Alzheimer's patients in America and 19 million of their family members grappling with issues surrounding their care. By the year 2050 there will be 14 million Americans diagnosed with AD if no cure or prevention is found.

Fading is a book that explores the debilitating nature of Alzheimer's disease from onset to death. My mother, Maxine A. Reinstein, aka, "Moose," had once been a prolific communicator. I have over 200 letters from her, spanning 30 years, that chronicle our family's life cycle events. She loved to write and talk. The catastrophic effects of this disease left her in a wheelchair muttering unintelligible sounds.

My heart broke each time I witnessed AD rob my mother of another ability. Scenes are etched in my memory that marked new lows. There was the time I arrived at her apartment to take her to lunch. She was waiting for me in the lobby clinging to an ice cream carton containing her wallet. And how can I forget when she confused lipstick for deodorant leaving her underarms a shocking ruby red? It was when language disappeared and I stared into her pleading brown eyes, knowing there was a person imprisoned there, that I felt most helpless. I was her link to the world – her lifeline – her voice. For this reason, I feel commissioned to write this book, to tell her story and make her voice heard. Her story is one of four million.

A person with AD can live from 3 to 30 years or more from onset of symptoms. Expenses increase as the disease progresses. Currently AD costs U.S. society at least $100 billion a year. Neither Medicare nor private health insurance covers the long term type of care most patients need. Seven out of ten AD patients live at home. Nearly 75% of the home care is provided by family and friends. The remainder is "paid" care costing an average of $12,500 per year. Families pay almost all of that out-of-pocket. *(Information provided by the Alzheimer's Association's Green-Field Library)*

I believe this book will be a helpful resource offering information on providing the best care in a most economical way. Although my mother lost the battle with AD, her last years were spent in a loving and active environment until the very end. We can help people do the same for their loved ones.

Chapter 1

THROUGH THE LOOKING GLASS

Placing the hotel key into the slotted opening, I felt like Alice about to enter another world thru the looking glass. A green light flashed signaling me to press the handle and open the door. On the other side of that door, I would come face to face with a long awaited journey into my past, a chronicle of my life presented through a collection of letters written to me by my mother. This chronicle would take me through passages I wasn't sure if I wanted to revisit. I saved these letters for 30 years with the promise to reread them upon my mother's death. Today was the 4th week anniversary of her passing and I was ready to embark on this adventure with mixed emotions.

It was imperative for me to do this without scheduling snafus and without considering anyone else's needs. I checked into the Broadmoor, a five-star hotel nestled in the foothills of Pikes Peak in Colorado Springs. The instructions to my family were simple, "Don't call." Although I travelled light with only an overnight bag and the bulging faux alligator attache case containing over 200 letters, the emotional baggage I carried was heavy.

My relationship with my mother had never been what I had wanted. That is, not until the end. My ideal mother would have been someone with whom I could share my inner-most thoughts, as well as, lighthearted afternoons of shopping, lunch and the theatre. Instead, I inherited a nervous, fearful and angry woman. I excused her behavior because she had suffered the loss of identical twins from which she never quite recovered. It was my brother's company and approval she sought, not mine. Yet, in the end, I was the one God appointed to escort her to death's door. He graciously gave me three years to repair my vision of what could have been and adjust to what was. In that time, resentment gave way to an abiding love that surpassed human understanding. I had forgiven my mother for not being my ideal. As the good book instructs us:

And become useful and helpful and kind to one another, tender-hearted, forgiving one another as God in Christ forgave you. Eph. 4:32

I checked into that hotel determined to rediscover my mother by check-out time. My only request, a room facing the mountains and lake, was granted. The windows and curtains were open affording commanding views of the Rockies. Muffled conversations and laughter of hotel guests below provided a touch of reality. It was dusk, my favorite time of day.

Settling myself next to the window, I picked up the first letter and something magical happened. I felt like I was reading it for the first time. Suddenly, I was transported back to 1974. My mother was a prolific writer, giving detailed accounts of events. She wrote like she spoke and I could hear her voice. Every letter was signed "Love, Moose," a nickname lovingly bestowed on her by my brother.

Amazingly, I didn't feel sad. Instead, I saw the richness of her life in terms of family connections –

spending holidays together, baby-sitting the grand children, and reunions with relatives at their large country lake home – a lifetime of togetherness that we were only privy to through her letters. My husband's military career took us to other parts of the country; Hawaii, San Francisco, Kansas and Colorado. But I could see how she yearned to have us be part of her world too. There were references to our forthcoming visits. The excitement of seeing us soon and wanting desperately to lavish attention on her absentee grandchildren was evident in her letters. Those letters emotionally tethered us to homebase.

The cast of characters has all but vanished. Aunts, uncles and friends were immortalized in Moose's letters. My life is a bit thinner without them all, but how grateful I am to her for those words painting intimate portraits of their interwoven lives. It was a three-dimensional story with me peeking through my mother's eyes.

The only time in two days I felt overcome by nostalgia was when incidents transcended generational lines. Things were discussed that spanned decades and linked us together like some invisible golden thread. Even minor things like reading about my grandmother making strawberry jam impacted me. I had just returned from Minnesota where my newly-married daughter and I had made strawberry jam.

I spent from 4:00 p.m. until 1:00 a.m. dancing through the years with my mother. I would have stayed up all night to be with her, but sleep overtook me. Already having read 50 letters, I still faced a huge stack. My sleep was restless. An overwhelming feeling that I had deserted her beckoned me back into her presence. She needed me. I awoke early, made a pot of coffee, brushed my teeth and jumped back into the past with

Moose. Hours passed as we revisited family crises like my father's stroke, critical surgeries, my brother's separation from his wife, triumphs, births, anniversaries, promotions and bar mitzvahs. In short, our family's life events were served on a silver platter for me to relive.

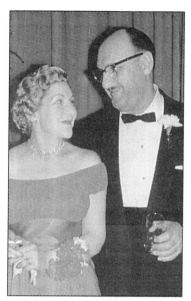

Moose and husband, Max, in the 1950's.

In this time, no great revelations occurred. What emerged was small pieces of her life that helped define her character and shed some light on what forged her relationships with others. After two days and nights, however, several themes surfaced. For example, there were at least a dozen references to the fact that Moose wanted my father to retire. He was a brilliant tax attorney losing his competitive edge. In lieu of retirement, my father opted to ignore several treatable health problems resulting in his death at 72. My mother had been his secretary for over 20 years and found herself suddenly husbandless and jobless. She kept his office open for a year, practicing law without a degree. My husband, Barry, a psychiatrist, always joked, "Thank goodness your father wasn't a surgeon."

Another reoccurring issue was weight. She was constantly writing about the latest diet fad guaranteeing a slim and happy life. If she gained four pounds, she let us know. The irony is that she died weighing less

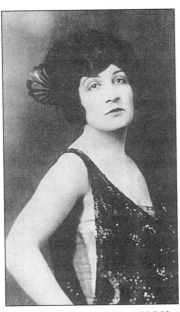
Madame Rose in the 1920's.

than 100 pounds. I share her weight struggle and pray that I will conquer this problem. By some miracle, my daughter has been able to sidestep this pothole. I could see my life as I read between the lines.

Despite the human frailties, the letters reveal how strong the women in my mother's family were. Her grandmother, Fanny, a German immigrant, managed to raise and educate five children. Rose, her only daughter, opened two hair salons at the age of 16 and was responsible for introducing the fingerwave to Chicago. She was referred to as Madame Rose in a Chicago Tribune article describing her contribution.

Later, she opened a jewelry store in the swanky Ambassador East Hotel. Her clientele included movie stars and future U.S. presidents. Although, diminutive in stature (standing only 4 feet, 11 inches), she was one tough business woman who raised two young daughters by herself during the depression and helped support four single brothers. Moose was constantly struggling to gain independence from her domineering mother, Madame Rose.

She complained often of doing things for friends and family members and not being appreciated for it. Moose was the consummate martyr. Her epistles were filled with lamentations about having to cook and clean

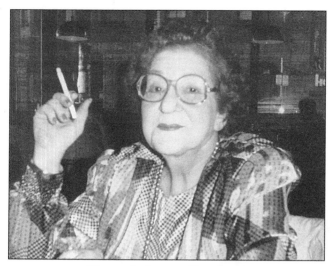
Moose in her earlier days.

for house guests, yet those very things made her feel useful. It was also, in a sense, how she expressed love. I can remember her agonizing over what she'd serve for lunch after finishing the breakfast dishes. I can count on one hand the number of times she retired her dishtowel to join us on the terrace for light banter. She lived in a beautiful home on a lake with a boat anchored outside and she elected to wash, cook and clean. I remember a family vacation in Florida where she spent her time washing clothes by hand and hanging them on the balcony as the rest of us lounged by the pool. It took me years to realize that she liked working for us and griping about it. That was her "MO" (military for "mode of operation").

Her relaxation was smoking a cigarette while doing a crossword puzzle. She claimed to love being with the family, but dedicated most of her time to serving and whining. If you offered to help with chores she'd refuse the assistance. When she was given gifts, she'd say, "Why did you spend the money on me?" She was-

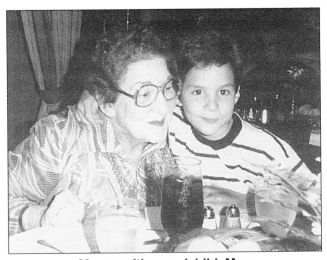
Moose with grandchild, Max.

n't particularly demonstrative except with the grandchildren. I always had to initiate any tenderness
between us. She just didn't know how to show her feelings. Somehow, I managed to perceive what she did for
me as loving. I appreciated her taking pains to write to
me in such graphic detail about life back home. In spite
of her human frailties, I grew to understand her.

Years later, in a conversation with a family friend,
she stated that the happiest times of her life were the
eight years she and my father spent at the lake house
commuting into Chicago. It was in that summer village,
Michiana, that they became active in local politics,
entertained family and friends and shared the richest
part of their life together. My father indulged his whims
with a 36 ft. cruiser. He would anchor the boat behind
the house and swim to shore for a lunch prepared by
my mother. To me, those were the Camelot years for the
entire family. It was there my husband, Barry, and I
married and returned with our children, Brandy and
Max, for reunions with the family. The times we shared

there left an indelible impression on me. Now in my early 50s, I long to reproduce that experience for my offspring. We had, in fact, purchased a lakeside home in the Ozarks, but sold it without having spent one day there because Moose was ill. Our dream would have to be put on hold.

My only regret is not saving the letters my mother wrote to me while I was attending college. They were classics. When one of her letters arrived at the sorority house, everyone would gather around as I read excerpts. They were filled with advice on a myriad of topics from how and when to empty my bladder to how I could avoid contracting the kissing disease (mononucleosis) by not going on coke dates. She had even mapped out which of the service stations enroute from Des Moines (where I attended Drake University) to Chicago, were clean enough to make my deposits. To this day, she is still quoted by some of my old college friends, as she advised me upon learning I would be spending the holidays with my roommate in Kentucky, "Empty your bladder, it's a long way to Louisville."

I was in my 40s and my mother still felt it necessary to give me a list of "moving tips," such as getting change of address cards from the post office, contacting the phone and utility companies, giving detailed instructions on how to pack my china, and etc.

For such an adroit communicator to be stricken with a disease that would reduce her to making incoherent animal like noises, there could be no worse fate. Her journey into silence compelled me to write on her behalf. I will say the words, I will tell her story.

This book is dedicated to Moose and all those whose memories have been erased and whose voices have been silenced by Alzheimer's Disease.

Chapter II

WHAT'S THE MATTER WITH MOOSE?

It was June of 1995, and it had become apparent that my mother's ability to live independently was diminishing. It took us by surprise since she had been an astute investor, doubling my father's estate, and had handled the sale of her Chicago condo without benefit of a realtor before relocating to Boca Raton, Florida.

We had asked my mother many times to live with us over the years, but she always wanted to maintain her independence, like her mother, who lived alone until her death at 90. Since she wouldn't come to us, we went to her – four times that year. Each time her behavior became more alarming making it difficult to take leave of her.

It began with delusions that mites were feasting on her internal organs. Then it spread to an infestation of mites in her furniture, causing her to sell brand new furniture at a fraction of its worth. From there the delusions transferred to people who were either stealing her money or out to kill her. My mother's conversations became peppered with violent overtones. She talked about how she was going to have a person "taken care of," or of her intent to throw a neighbor over the balcony for some perceived insult. As if all this weren't bad enough, her balance was being affected, causing her to take some serious falls on the street. In addition, her nutrition was suffering due to her poor diet.

them.

Right now I am being bitten by fleas. You can't see them; you only feel them bite you. My whole place is full of them. I am seriously thinking of going back to Skokie when my lease is up. I've had it!! I'll write again soon— I'm itching like crazy! Love ×××× Moose—"

An excerpt from one of Moose's letters.

On my third visit, there was no food in the house. My mother claimed to be on a canned soup diet. Instead of food, her refrigerator/freezer housed clothing and documents wrapped in plastic bags to prevent contamination from mites. I suspected that she had forgotten how to cook and soup was the easiest to prepare.

Least disconcerting, was the fact that a once articulate communicator was using words like "watchamacallit" or "thingamajig" to fill in for words that eluded her. Short and long term memory were impacted.

She had tried to discourage me from making this trip to check up on her. I think this was her defense mechanism to prevent me from discovering how bad her condition was. Undaunted, I had informed her several times of my travel arrangements and expected arrival time and reiterated the day before I was to travel. As I prepared to leave for the airport, I received a frantic call from her questioning why I was at home when she had expected me to arrive yesterday. She said she had called the police reporting me missing. She was irate and wouldn't listen to reason, hanging up on me. I don't cry easily, but, I sat on the edge of my bed, receiver in hand and became hysterical. My husband had to call her back and gently explain that the plans had always been for me to arrive that day.

She eventually relented, but the plane ride there was an anxious one for me. I had no idea how I'd be received. The blessing of this disease is that she forgot her anger and we had a wonderful time together.

Several months later, she called to say she had received her bank statement and noticed a check written to Sheryl, my sister-in-law, for $20,000, which she adamantly denied writing. This time, my husband, son and I boarded a plane determined to bring this to a conclusion. Either she would have to come back to Colorado with us or we would have to move to Florida. On this, our fourth trip, we came prepared to purchase a home near her, since she had refused all past offers to come back to Colorado and move in with us.

Since my last trip, my mother's balance became affected. She had fallen and to my knowledge had not gone to a doctor to check for possible injuries. Although she lived close to my brother, Reuben, he seemed inattentive to my mother's condition and now, it appeared that he was taking advantage of her financially.

After examining the signature on the $20,000 check, we concluded that it was identical to my mother's. At her insistence, we went to the bank and approached the man who normally handled her transactions. He said that he had, in fact, witnessed her signing this check. He said she came in that day with a middle-aged man and a younger man, fitting the description of my brother and nephew, who had become my mother's power of attorney that morning. As he was relating the events, he was writing on a note pad, which he shoved in my direction. It stated quite simply that my brother and nephew's plan was to deplete her funds and place her in a state home. I was horrified that they would even think of such a thing and then mystified that they would discuss it with a stranger. I felt compelled to show the note to my mother, who upon reading it, came out of her fog and looked at us and in a clear rational tone said, "Get me the hell outa here." This was a call to action.

A father of the fatherless and a judge and protector of the widows is God in His holy habitation. Psalm 68:5

God had used this messenger to reveal in a graphic way what my brother's plans held for our mother. What a mighty God we serve!

There is nothing concealed that will not be disclosed or hidden that will not be made known. Luke 12:2

Chapter III

THE GREAT ESCAPE

The shocking revelation of my brother's plan for her rocked my mother's world. Only then would she agree to move to Colorado with us. God seemed to clear the way. We had her packed up within four days with no interference from my brother. The realization that her son was conspiring to have her institutionalized was more than she could handle. Fearful of what he might do if he caught her in the act of dismantling her apartment, she moved into the hotel with us. She would sit on the edge of the bed holding her head and rocking. The only way she could cope was by blaming the situation on my sister-in- law. It was unbearable for her to conceptualize that the son, whom she had always favored, was capable of hatching such a plan. She spoke incessantly about buying him a divorce.

Before leaving the state, there were some legal issues we needed to handle. Since she would now be residing near us, we had to change the power of attorney from my nephew to me. We gathered all of the stock certificates that were strewn about my mother's apartment and took her to a brokerage firm we were familiar with to open an account for her. Our goal was to get her finances in order. There was a considerable amount of money missing, but it was impossible to trace what had happened to it. We could only speculate.

Once the moving trucks had departed with her belongings and we had taken care of loose ends, we were eager to leave Florida, as was she. Before our departure, I asked if she wanted me to call Reuben and advise him of her move to Colorado. She emphatically stated that she didn't want him to know of her whereabouts. I wrestled with this, but decided to honor her wishes. This would come back to haunt me.

Chapter IV

SETTLING IN

Considering the drama of it all, the move was without incident. Moose stayed with us for three weeks until we found her an apartment in a lovely retirement community. As long as we kept her focused on other things, she was okay. She likened the facility to a hotel because two meals were provided in a common dining room. It had a European feel to it, situated on a bluff overlooking the Rockies. Her corner apartment was pleasant with lots of light. The maintenance man lived directly across the hall, reassuring us that help was very accessible to her. There were many services provided, including a limo to take residents grocery shopping or to doctor's appointments. The staff was very friendly and helpful, making adjustments to accommodate the occupants who were mostly high functioning.

We knew her time there would be limited because of her increasing need for assistance, however, we committed to keeping her as independent as long as possible.

Everyday we would see her – sometimes twice a day. We'd share meals either at her "hotel" or at our home. It was wonderful having her so close by to make sure her needs were being met. One of the first tasks at hand was to have our family physician do a medical workup. He ran a battery of tests, including a cat scan and blood work to determine her general health. When we went to pick up her medical records from her physician, he said that he hadn't seen her in several years. It was no surprise, given her "soup diet," that amongst other things she was suffering from malnutrition. The scan revealed that there was significant shrinkage and calcium deposits in her brain, indicating Alzheimer's Disease. She was prescribed a new memory enhancing drug and an anti-delusional medication to try, although all talk of mites had already ceased.

Once we got a handle on her medical condition, we could pay attention to some other areas, i.e., getting appropriate clothing for the winter months. I was appalled at the condition of her undergarments, many being frayed or torn. She was a woman of means and didn't need to be denying herself anything. Shopping with her was fulfilling a fantasy of mine which was having a normal mother/daughter relationship, whiling away the hours in department stores and "doing lunch." Even in her diminished capacity it was fun having input on how she should dress. It was my pleasure to buy her neat hats and accessories. For me, it was like re-creating her into the mom I'd always yearned to have.

At last my children were benefiting from having a grandparent nearby. Because of Barry's military career, we never had the privilege of living close to relatives. We lived vicariously enjoying holidays spent with other people's families. It was fun having her over for dinner. I especially enjoyed even the most mundane things, like watching her set the table while I prepared dinner, as the kids played their loud music. Our dinner conversations consisted of filling in the blanks for her as she lost more and more vocabulary. I felt fulfilled and honored to be able to assist my mother in this stage of her life.

Exodus 20:12 entreats us to **Honor thy father and mother**. My family was living out that commandment.

Laced with the richness of adding a new dimension to our lives (caring for my mother), was an ever-present feeling of sadness. Each time we reached a new plateau representing the loss of another of my mother's skills, I grieved. Poignant scenes stand out in my mind; the time I arrived at her "hotel" for lunch to find her sitting in the lobby, clutching an ice cream carton with her wallet in it, the day she mistakenly used lipstick for deodorant, and the moment we realized she'd forgotten how to use her key? I can recall how Moose would pace the floor at our house, examining every inch, claiming she had

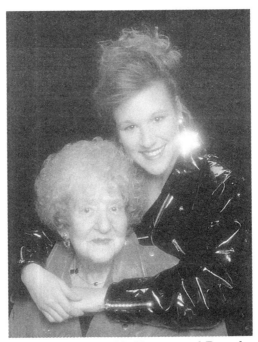

Glamour photo with Moose and Brandy soon after Moose moved to Colorado.

made and installed the carpeting. She would repeatedly say, "This is mine."

The saddest for me was a story my daughter related. I had out of town guests I hadn't seen in years who were coming for dinner. Only Moose and I were home. In the middle of roasting the lamb, my oven blew a coil. Moose was excitedly telling my daughter, Brandy, about our mishap. She tried very hard to think of the word "oven." Brandy began the "word-guessing game" to complete my mother's thought. Finally, with tears in her eyes, Moose turned away and said, "Never mind." It was these times that she recognized her waning ability to communicate that disturbed me the most. We would try to make light of it as best we could. I knew there would come a day when she may not even recognize me. All we could do was take it a day at a time.

So do not worry or be anxious about tomorrow, for tomorrow will have worries and anxieties of its own. Sufficient for each day is its own trouble. Matthew 6:34

Chapter V

THE DILEMMA

Moose was with us a month, when we decided to go on a business trip. We would be gone for 2-3 weeks and I desperately wanted Moose to come with us. We were having trouble adjusting her medication and wanted to monitor it.

Her behavior took a turn. We were under the impression that the delusions were over since she no longer spoke of mites. However, now we had become part of her delusions. Missing my brother and his family, she called him. Apparently, in order to justify leaving so abruptly, she told him we had kidnapped her and brought her to Colorado. I knew something was up because every time we came to her apartment she would have a scowl on her face and act very suspicious of us. She refused to come with us on the trip. Reluctantly, we left, but not before we had a network of support people in place to call and look in on her. I spoke to her banker and stock broker telling them I suspected she might be up to something and to not allow her to withdraw any large sums of money.

We called her daily as well as having people check in on her. Each person expressed grave concerns because she was telling everyone we were trying to kill her and had brought her to Colorado against her will. She mentioned to one friend that she had called a detective to press charges against us and that we were going to be arrested when we arrived home. Her delusions were alive and well!

My brother, unfortunately, was feeding into them. I'm sure from his perspective what she was saying all made sense. After all, his mother leaves Florida without a trace and without so much as a good-bye. When we were packing her up to leave Florida, I asked if she wanted me to call Reuben to notify him we were taking her back to Colorado. It was at her insistence that he not be told where she was. She even instructed her sister, my aunt Lucille, not to divulge her whereabouts in the event Reuben called making inquiries. I was in a bind.

I wondered, do I honor my mother's request against my better judgment, or let him draw his own conclusions? This dilemma was so upsetting I sought the counsel of our pastor, who advised, "As long as your mother is still able to make decisions regarding her welfare, you honor her."

Needless to say, all throughout our trip I was petrified of the outcome. Would we arrive home to find the police on our doorstep? Would pictures of us being taken away in handcuffs be blasted all over the front page of *The Gazette*? How would our friends react if we were arrested on kidnapping charges? As usual, God was in control and I needn't have worried.

After our return, I called the detective my mother had mentioned to a friend she had contacted. He assuaged our fears by telling us that the police would have been on our doorstep if they had thought there was even a grain of truth to the story. He further stated that if anyone intended to kidnap a person they wouldn't place them in an apartment with access to a phone and the freedom to escape. Finally, and most importantly, he said, "If your brother was so concerned, why didn't he hop on a plane to assess your mother's situation like you people did when you realized your mother was having difficulty in Florida?" I was flooded with relief.

Our problems didn't end there. Moose's delusions were at full tilt and she refused to let us near her. We called social services to enlist their help in getting her properly diagnosed. It was then that I realized she needed to be declared incompetent and a court appointed conservator, a neutral party, had to step in to handle her finances, given the estrangement between my brother and I. A social worker was sent to her apartment for an interview. There was little she could do unless Moose was a danger to herself or others, or if she would voluntarily enter a hospital with a diagnostic unit. It was agony being separated from her, not knowing what she would do. We'd call her and she would scream at us and hang up the phone. I notified everyone around her to be on the alert for any bizarre behavior.

Chapter VI

MOOSE ON THE LOOSE

An answer to prayer came one day with a phone call from the maintenance man from Moose's apartment. He informed us that Moose had called a taxi and was intending to run away. Thanking him profusely, I instructed him to stall her while we called the cab company and arranged to have her taken to the hospital and held for observation. We called the hospital that had a diagnostic unit and arranged to have personnel greet the cab and admit my mother immediately. We had to stay in the background fearing she would become violent upon seeing us. Everything went according to plan, except that my mother was able to convince the cab driver her story was true. He struggled with allowing the hospital staff to escort her to a locked ward. After a few minutes he backed off and my mother was led away into the hospital without incident.

The hardest thing about putting her in the hospital was being separated from Moose physically and emotionally. She wanted nothing to do with us. We were , however, relieved to know she was in good hands and safe. With professional help, the situation would be brought under control. We went up to the ward to observe her. I worried about her mental condition. Was she frightened? How would she adjust to being in a locked ward of a hospital? These questions plagued me. The staff told us she was doing rather well and was able to eat. God bless her, nothing affected her appetite!

Over the next week, we met with a psychologist, a court appointed attorney, social workers, doctors, etc. Moose was given a full battery of tests to assess her daily living skills and determine if she was capable of handling her own affairs. In the meantime, she was put on medication to control delusions. The hope was that when the medicine kicked in, she would not remember being so angry and fearful toward us. She did agree to see the kids, Brandy and Max. We sent them with her favorite candy, coloring books and flowers. Delighted to see a familiar face, she embraced them wholeheartedly. We prayed that these feelings would eventually include Barry and I.

I was informed that I would have to serve my mother with papers calling for a competency hearing. This was the hardest thing I have ever had to do. My consolation was that I knew this had to be done and the blessing of this disease was that she would forget all about how angry she was with me. There was nothing I wanted more than to hold her and reassure her that all would be okay.

After one week, the medication took affect. Moose, seeing Barry at the nurse's station, smiled and motioned him to come in to see her. It seemed a miracle of miracles. Barry was back to being her beloved son-in-law and not some kidnapper! He asked if she would like to see me and she said, "Of course." I was elated. Later that day, we all went to see her and had a very nice visit. She would be released at the end of the week and some plans had to be in place as to how we could insure the best living arrangements.

We met with the staff who had her test results in hand. They had informed her that she would be needing help daily to which she was quite agreeable. I was appointed her medical guardian, able to make all decisions regarding her general health. I was also to take control of her finances until a conservator could be selected.

There were court dates set for all of us to meet with a judge, the court appointed guardian, my brother, via telephone, and Moose herself. A gentleman named Kenny Levitt was chosen to handle my mother's financial affairs. Kenny was no stranger. We had traveled in some of the same social circles and I felt he could be trusted. The judge ordered a complete assessment of Moose's estate. It was a relief to turn over all the files I had gathered. From the time she had moved to Colorado I had worked, with the help of a broker, to get her finances in order. It was a tremendous responsibility.

The entire process of turning Moose's life over to the courts and structuring a system dedicated to her well-being, took about four months.

Chapter VII

HELP IS ON THE WAY

In addition to Moose's financial affairs, there was also the question of getting assistance with life skills, such as bathing, dressing and taking medication. The goal was to keep her living independently, in her apartment, as long as it was feasible.

One of the maids at my mother's complex had a daughter, Angelique, who was experienced in elder care. We hired her to come in three times daily, to help my mother with laundry, light house cleaning and tending to her personal care. My mother accepted all of the changes in her life graciously, without argument. On some level I suspect she was relieved to have her affairs taken care of. Alzheimer's patients go through such tumult when they are aware enough to know things aren't as they should be. It is not unusual to find hundreds of scraps of papers with notes and numbers in their apartments as they struggle to maintain control of their lives. Angelique was employed for about 2 months and would be the first of many care givers.

We hit another of those devastating plateaus when one day I phoned my mother and she said she didn't know why, but she was all wet. Angelique wasn't there. I dashed right over to see what the problem was and found that my mother had become incontinent. This began a new phase entailing diapers. Now, Angelique would have to check on my mother at noon and dinner time to make sure she had not soiled herself before she would go down to eat a meal. I didn't want her to embarrass herself.

I can vividly recall several times when I would arrive at Moose's to check up on her (since she now had forgotten how to use the phone and couldn't call me when she needed something) and find feces all over her and the chairs. I knew she probably had tried to clean herself up. God gave me the strength to handle the situation without ever feeling disgusted with my mother. I would always try to maintain her dignity, and reassure her it was okay.

I have strength for all things in Christ Who empowers me. Phil. 4:13

Before long we discovered that Angelique was taking advantage of the situation by billing us for time she wasn't putting in. One day, Kenny, the conservator, arrived at my mother's apartment to give Moose the weekly allowance, and he discovered Angelique asleep on my mother's sofa. That was the clincher. As soon as I could find a replacement, Angelique would be history. My mother no longer was able to occupy her time; she couldn't turn on the television, write a letter or use the phone without assistance. Also, she had begun to fall more frequently. More hours would be required of Angelique's replacement.

One afternoon, after Angelique had gone to the dining room to get my mother's lunch, Moose ran to get the phone and fell. I was at a shower for a friend's daughter-in-law when I received a phone call from my husband informing me of the fall and asking me to meet him at the emergency room. We waited a long time until the doctor came back with the X-ray results indicating there were no broken bones. That was the last day of my mother's independence. We moved her in with us that evening. It also marked the end of Angelique's employment with us.

Chapter VIII

IN THE TRENCHES

Once my mother moved in with us, we were on the front lines with no time for ourselves. There was no hiding place, and no escape. We were on duty 24/7. This elicited a bundle of feelings in having to deal with situations that strained our patience. The following are excerpts from a journal I began to keep:

Sometimes I feel so frustrated, I could scream and shake her, but I know she is equally frustrated with me. The difficult times are when she can't find a place for herself, generally late afternoon. I'm told this is the sundown syndrome, where the Alzheimer's patient believes they should be at home taking care of their family. 'Home' meaning the town they lived in either as a youth or where they raised their children. She gets up, paces, and sits back down countless times. She looks at me as if to say 'can't you do something?' I try to engage her in some activity, like helping prepare dinner or setting the table, but she can only be distracted for a little while. The doctors are at a loss for how to treat this. My knight in shining armor is Barry, who, seeing when I am about ready to blow, offers to take Mother for a ride in the car. She loves the car and like a child, is often lulled to sleep by the motion, or just sits quietly taking in the scenery. I am so grateful for that time alone when they are gone.

Another annoying behavior that emerged was Moose asking to go to the bathroom, getting in there and then forgetting why she was there. It seems like every 10 minutes she's asking to go in the bathroom again. Barry thinks perhaps it is one of the areas she still had control over or that she is so afraid of being incontinent she wants to make sure there are no "accidents". Sometimes, I just pray God will take her before it becomes too bad. I don't know how long I'll be able to take this.

Then there are the funny times. She can be a little lamb. When we are walking she holds my hand and calls me mother. Talk about a reversal of roles! Her hand feels frail in mine like a child's, so dependent and trusting. We were recently at a restaurant where the service was particularly slow. The waitress said, "Your food will be out shortly."

My mother quickly retorted, "Yeah, sure." There is something freeing about her condition because she can say anything she pleases and no one takes offense.

There was the time I had scheduled her to go to Namnaste, a day program for adults, so she could have more to do during the day other than falling asleep in front of the television. I tried to prepare her for the day saying she would be less bored being with people her own age. The night before I reminded her she would be going. She was adamant about not going. I felt like I was dealing with a five-year-old before her first day of kindergarten. After a long, animated conversation with my children present, I decided to drop it. She had every right to be bored. I needed to let her make some decisions regarding her own life.

My mother's one real pleasure is listening to Barry and Max rehearse with their '50s singing group, "Now and Then." She is their number one fan, attending every performance. The lead singer, John, will come over and hold her hand and sing to her. He made her feel very special.

One evening, after the group had performed at the Broadmoor Hotel, she had a far away look in her eyes as we were preparing her for bed. Brandy asked her what she was thinking about and she replied, "I wonder if I could have a career in singing?"

I thought this was precious, that she could still dream. We asked if she remembered any songs. She said, "No."

I said, "Can you sing 'Da, da, da'?" We proceeded to practice *Call Me Irresponsible*, using the word "da" to fill in. It gave us all hope. Here my mother was in an advanced stage of Alzheimer's, believing with our encouragement that she could still have dreams for the future.

May the God of your hope so fill you with all joy and peace in believing that by the power of the Holy Spirit you may abound and be overflowing with hope. Romans 15:13

There were many wonderful, memorable times like when she came with me to a Bikers For Jesus meeting. All these tough looking guys with long hair and tattoos wearing leather, welcomed Moose in her walker with open arms. Months later we were at a Cinco de Mayo celebration in the park where the singing group performed, and the president of the Bikers club called out, "Hey, Moose! It's me, Penguin."

Our friends have been very supportive always remembering to include Moose in their invitations to us. They listened to me pour out my frustrations. We began

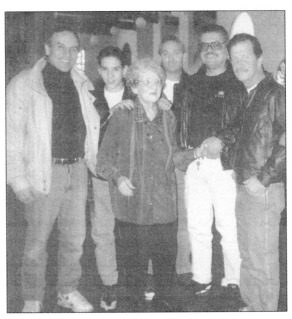

Moose with band members of *Now and Then*.

entertaining more at home with pot luck dinners or an evening of Scrabble. We brought activity into the home.

On her 81st birthday we celebrated at the temple where I got her involved with the senior lunch program. I had ordered a cake with a moose on it. Barry's singing group performed publicly for the first time. John sang songs directly to Moose and Barry asked her to get up and dance in front of everyone. She felt like a queen. I don't know if she had ever received so much attention, even from my father. That night we took her to dinner at the Broadmoor Hotel.

Sometimes I just sit and watch her while she naps. I think, "That can't be my mother, once so vibrant, now so frail. She looks like my grandmother. Worse yet, if she is my mother, looking so old, how old do I look?" When I pass a mirror, the vision of myself as a 25-year-old in my head is betrayed by the reflection of a middle-aged over weight woman. I detest seeing her so old and vulnerable. I'm relieved when she sleeps. She looks peaceful and I have free time. When she's awake, there are demands – mostly bathroom or feeding duties. Yet, she is always willing to go on an outing. She never turns down an opportunity to go.

There were times as I was growing up and developing a sense of who I was and wanted to be, that I was ashamed of my mother because she wore cheap clothes. She prided herself on the bargains she got while shopping in the basements of major department stores. I grew up thinking there were only two floors to a store - the main and basement. When I was old enough to shop and pay for my own clothes, I loved to dress well. Even though her mother owned a classy jewelry store at the ritzy Ambassador East Hotel, Moose delighted in wearing cheap plastic jewelry. The biggest coup of her life was buying 10 strands of colorful plastic beads for a buck a piece.

When she came to Colorado, we went shopping for new clothes and accessories. It was ironic that as she lost control of her life and became dependent, even to the point where she couldn't wipe her own bottom, in my eyes she was never more regal or beautiful. Finally, I had become proud of her. My instructions to her caregivers always included this statement, "My mother is a beautiful woman. I want her silvery-white curly hair always combed and make-up on her face." I would pay a beautician friend of mine to come and do my mother's hair and nails. Her skin was nearly flawless with very few wrinkles. Everyone meeting her for the first time would comment about her complexion. She had aged beautifully. I bought her crystal beads and matching

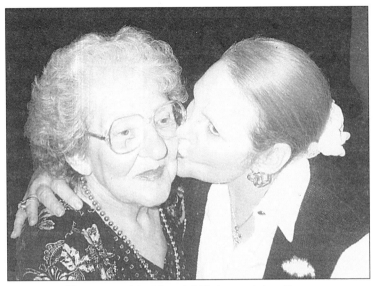

Moose and I at her birthday celebration.

earings from Austria. She loved to wear them when going out. I'd ask, "Do you want to wear the 'crown jewels' tonight?" I saw to it that she always looked nice and well groomed.

It always bothered me that Moose wouldn't spend money on herself and her clothes or appearance, even though money was not a problem for her. I can see now how much of who I am is a result of not wanting to be like her. I had worked for Barbizon Modeling School after sending myself through their school to develop my own sense of fashion style. I was unable to learn from my mother. I also saw to it that my daughter went to modeling school to learn how to enhance her looks. It was important that I provided my daughter with a good role model since I pretty much had to figure things out for myself.

There were the not-so-pleasant times also, when, for example, Moose would tell off a guest in our home for some small offense. One Sunday, my son had a friend over. He was a very tall boy diagnosed with Marphan's disease. For some reason his height bothered my mother. I had gone out with my daughter and upon returning home, received a report that she not only yelled at Max's friend, but when the mother came to pick him up she yelled, "Get out." Max was visibly upset and it struck an all too familiar cord in me.

As a teenager, I recall my grandmother, Rose, hanging up on my friends when they would call for me in addition to making some rude remark. I knew I had to curtail this behavior because hostessing was one of my strong suits and I never wanted anyone feeling uncomfortable in my home. I told my mother she had no business treating Max's friend so rudely. She responded, "It's me or them."

I told her she needed to make other living arrangements then because being rude to our friends would not be tolerated in our home. Moose had enough sense remaining to keep quiet. We proceeded to go out for dinner and have a nice evening. The hidden blessing in this disease is that you can forget what has been said or done moment to moment. That incident evoked such strong memories from my childhood about my grandmother embarrassing me and my mother not interceding on my behalf, that this was one place for me to change the script. I was going to take a strong stand and protect my children from any further embarrassing behavior.

It was often difficult to determine how much negative behavior was attributable to the disease and how much was just my mother. Whenever it was clear that it was the disease causing my mother to act a certain way, I would appeal to the children and ask them to have mercy. Particularly, when Moose became violent trying to hit, bite and scratch as they were lifting her. I knew my mother was never prone to that kind of outburst and would ask whoever it was directed at to forgive her and ignore it.

The most powerful and overriding emotion I felt at any time was pride and love for my family as I watched them individually treat my mother with honor and respect. I had promised my mother I would never put her in a home. This was my commitment to her. I also felt bound by the commandment *"**Honor thy father and mother.**"* I felt that this was my most compelling calling in life; to escort my mother to her death with dignity intact. I never expected this unending, unwavering support and commitment from my children and husband. If I thought I loved my husband 22 years ago when we recited our vows, it was nothing compared to what I felt when I was told he had cleaned her and her bowel movement up from the kitchen floor.

When I saw my children lovingly escort my mother to and from the car, in and out of restaurants and to the bathroom, my heart was exploding with pride. I knew I was modeling for them how I wanted to be treated if I was ever in my mother's condition some day. Nothing could compare to the feeling I had when strangers would comment in public places what a wonderful family we were because of the light we were giving off. I feel we were a beacon to many in this day and age when so many people warehouse their elderly family members in homes when they become too troublesome.

One incident remains indelibly etched in my mind. It was my 51st birthday and we chose to celebrate quietly, just the five of us. We went to a small rustic restaurant in the mountains called the Swiss Chalet. We ate outside as it was a typically beautiful summer's evening and my favorite time of day, dusk. The mountains were silhouetted against a darkening deep purple sky. Our conversation was animated, as usual, when we all came together, filled with humor, joking, topic skipping and sharing. We loved to share entrees so food was being passed all around the table. I couldn't help but notice a woman dining alone. I knew she was listening to our conversation because she would smile at things we were saying. As we were leaving, Max and Brandy were walking my mother, and Barry and I were trailing behind. The woman stopped us and said, "You have a wonderful family. I wanted you to know how much I enjoyed watching all of you. It is obvious you are a close loving family. How lucky you are." This was not an isolated incident. It was as if God was sending us love notes. These times were so rich and filled with meaning.

I also remember the morning my mother awoke at 4 a.m. and was ready to start the day. After much gentle persuasion, I returned her to bed, but decided to stay up and journal. Barry was awake so I asked if he wanted to read what I had written. Shortly afterward, the

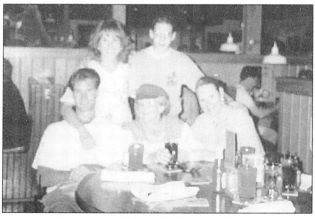

Moose, out to eat with all of us.

bedding erupted into volcanic-sized shaking and I realized he was weeping. For the first time, we both lay side by side crying. When we composed ourselves again, I asked what in particular moved him. All he said was, "It's good, very, very good." I guess putting into words what we were all feeling and experiencing was cathartic.

At one point, I started attending support groups offered by the local Alzheimer's Association. The topics were always timely such as "Stress On Caregivers to Alzheimer's Patients" or "Appropriate Placement Alternatives." The most beneficial part was hearing from other caregivers on how they dealt with issues. I needed this organization as they offered tremendous support.

I was most appreciative when Barry, recognizing I needed relief, would say to Mother, "Come on Moose, let's just you and me go for a ride," or "Let's go to breakfast, Moose, just the two of us." There was so much emotional outlay surrounding my mother's care that I didn't have much left for anything or anybody else. I felt I was only on the receiving end with them. How I relished that time alone.

I soon realized that because of the additional time needed for my mother, other areas were suffering, i.e. housecleaning. Days would go by with chores only half completed; silverware from a dinner party from weeks ago waiting to be put away, laundry piled up, dead flowers in a vase, dust collecting on a glass table. I forgave myself for this conspicuous neglect and decided to enlist the help I needed whatever the cost. The additional strain of going through this without benefit of talking to my estranged brother, saddened me.

My mother was a great movie partner. She loved the cool, dark theater and much to my surprise, she stayed awake and alert. She really loved action films and like a child, demanded candy. After all, what's a good movie without something to accompany it?

For me, it was a great escape to forget my woes for two hours giving me the interlude I needed to deal with reality. We also took Moose to plays, state fairs, etc. She led a more well-rounded life than ever before. She loved my son's preference for rock and roll and didn't care how loud he cranked up the car radio. We'd say, "Come on Moose, shake your booty," and she would shimmy her shoulders and get a cute impish smile on her face. She could be absolutely delightful.

I'll never forget the period when she thought that by cashing a $20 bill for four $5's or two $10's, she was making money. It began one evening when we went for pizza. She handed me a $20 bill to pay and when I returned with her change, she was ecstatic thinking she had made money! That was the beginning of a ritual between us. She would give me a few 20's and instruct me to go get her some more money. I would return with stacks of fives, tens or ones. She'd say, "Why aren't more people making money this way?" This continued for several months. I'd run all over town cashing 20's for her, but the inconvenience was worth the childlike pleasure she received. At one point, she handed my friend a $20 bill and said, "Here, I want to start you on the way to becoming a millionaire. Just ask Fran where to take this to get more money."

My mother was not cheap. She had a sense of fairness and would offer to treat us to a meal once in a while, recognizing that we had been good to her. She always tried to be equitable. After paying my sister-in-law's tuition to graduate school, she sent me a $10,000 bond to even the score, a score she kept track of. This sense of fairness never left her. She was grateful and showed it.

After a few months living with us, we entered a new phase. Moose began disrobing. She would apparently get up early, 4 a.m. or so, get undressed and come upstairs in the dark to our bedroom wearing only panties. One such morning, Barry and Moose met in the kitchen both were stark naked. Shocked at seeing each other, they broke out into hysterical laughter.

On several occasions, when we arose in the morning, Moose was nowhere to be found. We would usually find her sitting in the car parked in the garage, naked. Fortunately, she had not figured out how to exit the house by herself, or we may have found her roaming the neighborhood in her "all together." It is fascinating that none of these phases lasted too long, several months at the most. It is akin to a child passing through certain developmental stages that seem intolerable and disappear just when you think you can't stand another minute of it.

One of the physical side effects of Moose's medication was a tremor around her mouth and a shuffling gait. We would remind her, "Take big steps." Barry would say, "Stop walking like a Chinese woman whose feet have been bound." She still had an acute sense of humor with an ability to laugh at herself and circumstances.

I dreaded the day when she would no longer be able to speak. I also agonized over the inevitability that we would become unrecognizable to her. Everything was referred to as "watchamacallit," as she struggled to find the intended word. We knew her stories so well that we could fill in the blanks. Still, there were many times when she became so frustrated, as did we, when we couldn't guess what she was trying to say.

Chapter IX

PATIENCE IS AN EIGHT LETTER WORD

At this point in our journey with Moose, a friend, who is a Christian author, recommended I date my journal entries to track the progress of the disease. Admittedly, I was not faithful in my entries, but managed to capture some of our struggles.

8/21/96 *Today was the first day Moose wandered out of the house. I could vaguely hear someone walking around at 6 a.m. When I got up, I couldn't find her anywhere. The garage door was slightly ajar indicating she may have gone outside. Lo and behold! There she was sitting in the car, naked. She was very restless and nothing seemed to calm her – even after Anna* (the caretaker at that time) *came at 7 a.m. to get her washed and dressed. Today she seems particularly unsettled. She had a bowel movement but wouldn't stay on the toilet to finish. After cleaning her up she wanted to sit back on the toilet. I tried explaining that she needed to stay on the toilet until she completed the job. This little exercise continued for quite awhile until I had to pull the remaining feces from her rectum with baby wipes and toilet paper. This was not how I wanted to spend the day! I had to use the plunger to dispose of the waste.*

I'm angry at her and my brother, who doesn't even bother to visit her. Sometimes, I get so pent up with emo-

tion, I forget to breathe and my stomach hurts.

At these times I feel I need a tranquilizer to make it through. My nerves are shot. I'll go read the Bible in the hopes I can get relief or peace.

8/29 I'm losing my mother in pieces. It seems that each day she becomes a little more impaired. This disease is like a thief who takes his time robbing you of one treasure at a time.

8/31 I awoke at 4 a.m., frightened. It was the child in me scared of losing my mother and being all alone. There is still no one as much in my corner as she is. She always rushes to my defense if the kids or Barry get on my case. It is reminiscent of the time my in-laws came to visit and invited us to go swimming at the hotel. Nothing was more unappealing to me than to appear in a swimsuit 50 pounds heavier, complete with cellulite and spider veins. My mother, as if reading my mind, said, "Go ahead you're a great swimmer and you are beautiful." That kind of support was hard to resist. I changed into my suit and my mother, from the sidelines, gave me a very frail thumbs-up sign. Wow!

9/1 Labor Day. We went on two picnics (Sunday and Monday) and had a good time. We went to a double feature movie. Moose couldn't sit through the second movie so my dear husband, sensing I wanted to stay, said, "Come on Moose, let's you and me have a date. We'll go to dinner." They were waiting for us when the movie was over. While they were dining, several people we knew came up to them. Moose said, "I wonder what they will think of the two of us being together without your wife." There were so many moments like this to chuckle over.

Chapter X

ENTER: THE GIRLS

9/5 *God sent us two "angels" named Rosie and Tammy. They referred to themselves as "the girls." Barry met them just after they stopped working in a retirement home. They left because of the abuse (to the patients) they witnessed. They were in need of work and liked older people. They were willing to do light house work and also do crafts with Moose. The timing couldn't have been more perfect. Anna, Moose's current aide, had to leave because her baby was due. Barry and I had a business meeting in Denver, Brandy had a class and Max had a friend sleeping over. The girls would watch Moose. I did not want the children to be burdened with caring for my mother. They needed to have as normal a life as possible.*

Just before the girls had arrived to watch Moose the previous night, Moose was in a tizzy because Max was having a friend over, so Barry took her for a ride. I had reached my limit with her and was grateful for the time alone to get ready. I was looking for a pair of nylons, when I saw two notes Moose had written and given to us a few months earlier. One was to Barry thanking him for driving her places, and instructing him to keep singing and stay healthy. The note to me expressed her gratitude to me for all that I was doing and said, "Something good was sure to happen," to me. She, in fact, had taken out a $10,000 bond due on her death. Tears came flooding down my cheeks. I realized that the cranky woman I had just lost patience with, was not my mother. These two letters jogged my memory that my mother had thanked us in advance, even though she was now unable to express herself.

When we arrived home from our business meeting, there was a perfectly painted ceramic Santa Claus that Moose had created. She was quite the artist! The next morning when she arose, we raved about her art work. I saw a light go on. She was excited and so was I.

9/6 *The five of us went to Andrew Lloyd Weber's Music of the Night, a musical review of his Broadway plays. We all enjoyed it, especially Moose. It prompted memories of music in her life. She spoke about playing piano by ear, her father singing along as she played and her mother refusing to pay for any more lessons because she wouldn't practice. For the first time in a long time she was talkative and happy.*

9/7 *It was a beautiful morning and I wanted to take my mother to the Farmer's Market. I thought she would enjoy walking around, seeing the colorful fruits and vegetables on the backs of the truck along with all the booths for crafts. Max came with.*

9/20 *I awoke early, before dawn, today. The feeling of isolation was overpowering. With the exception of a few people,I don't feel a lot of support from friends now. I find this extremely hurtful because of all the times we've been there for others. My tendency, anyway, is to withdraw when there is a perceived hurt on my part. Because this disease, by it's very nature, isolates your loved one as communication wanes, it's easy to withdraw as well. I see it happening. My mother barely speaks intelligently* *anymore. There are often almost no recognizable words coming out. It sounds like gibberish. I'm forced into guessing what it is she is trying to say. Now, as we drive around town, there are greater silences. It's easier for me to not attempt talking to her because silence has become a relief compared to the frustration of trying to have a conversation. There is still a light in her eyes. I want sometimes to retreat with her into that black hole and rescue her – but from what?*

Today it feels like the black hole is a safer place to be insulating me from a world where very few people really care. Because this disease doesn't have a dramatic ending, just a slow fading away, people tend to think you are not mourning, bit by bit, the losses you experience. It makes me draw closer to my family and you, God, who are always there. It's light out now with no sign of my mother and I think, Oh God, is this the day she won't wake up? Then I hear Barry saying, "Good morning Moose," and I think I have her another day. Thank you God, for every day.

9/22 *What a miracle! I was getting dressed to go to church and Moose asked where I was going. When I answered, "Church," she said, "Can I come?" Wow! After a year and a half of her moving to Colorado and inviting her, she has requested to come. I know God is at work here. He can meet us at any level or age. He touched Max at age five so that he could understand and accept His truth, why couldn't He reach Moose at 82?*

9/29 *On Friday, I had purchased tickets for a "Night of Gershwin" concert presented by the symphony. We had dinner out with the Bichsels (the parents of*

Brandy's boyfriend, Dirk). We had box seats. Moose seemed thrilled to hear the guest pianist perform "Rhapsody In Blue." I got a kick out of watching her clap her hands so delicately and at one point she looked at me and smiled and I knew I had done something good for her. It felt like we had made a deep connection without a word spoken between us. We both shared a love of Gershwin, all this conveyed with one smile. Afterward we left the auditorium and Max was pushing Moose in the wheelchair. He loves jumping on the back of the chair and popping wheelies, all the while pretending he is driving a car. It was a little too wild a ride for her and she didn't hesitate to complain. So Max said, "Hey, you have it easy, just sitting there and riding around." We all laughed. It was a wonderful evening.

9/30 *Moose came to church again. We didn't ask we just got her dressed. Here's another blessing, Tammy, Rosie and Rosie's brother, Alan have been coming to our little church in the woods. That is so gratifying. When they came to get Moose ready, she was somewhat undressed. Rosie said, "Hey Moose, we can't have you walking around like that, there's a man out here (referring to her brother, Alan)." Moose quipped when asked what she thought she was doing and said, "I'm trying to get fan mail." We all burst out laughing. There is still a trace of her wit intact.*

9/30 *Later - I just experienced a myriad of feelings. I had a fight with Barry over nothing. I'm angry to be losing my last parent. I can run the gamut of emotions – self-pity, anger, sorrow, etc., in the space of a few minutes.*

Chapter XI

GOOD THINGS HAPPEN TOO

10/21 It has been weeks since my last entry. So much has happened in this period. We had invited Dirk's family, the Bichsels, over for a traditional Jewish Shabbat dinner. We felt it was important to share our Jewish heritage with them, even though our mutual love of Jesus had already bonded us.

I had been preparing for weeks; shopping, cooking, cleaning and putting gold decals on my good dinner dishes so I could set the table with my finest. There were fresh cut flowers and scented candles strategically placed around the house. The girls helped me cook special Jewish dishes like chopped liver, matzo ball soup, noodle kugel, strudel and brisket.

The night before the dinner, Dirk surprised Brandy by asking her to marry him and presenting her with a ring. The next morning, he arrived at our home with a bouquet of flowers and asked Barry and I for our permission to wed our daughter. Our Shabbat dinner turned into a wonderful celebration. The air was charged with emotion as I lit the Shabbat candles and recited the blessing, welcoming the Sabbath.

This was a blending of two families with Barry and Dirk's father, Stan, each taking their rightful positions at the head of the table. Everything I had prepared came out perfect. It was as if God's hand was on this union. We were all kvelling (Yiddish for "swelling with pride") and swept away by the moment.

The following day, Dirk and his mother, Barbara, brought us a beautiful flowering plant. Love was in bloom and so was our house!

10/22 After recovering from the initial shock, I sprang into high gear planning the event we dreamed of for so long. It was like trying to wade through alligator infested waters to avoid offending someone. Barry's parents were very sensitive about what kind of ceremony would be held, because while we had embraced Christianity, they did not share our beliefs. Barry called them to ask for the list of relatives they thought we should invite. They replied, "Nobody, and we're not coming either." Barry responded, "Well, that makes it clear as to who should not be sent invitations." They wanted to know where it would be held and who would officiate. Barry said, "Whether it's held in a church, hotel or synagogue, there will be much mentioned about Jesus, since that is what we believe in." The conversation ended shortly after that statement.

The bride-to-be came into her father's office and we

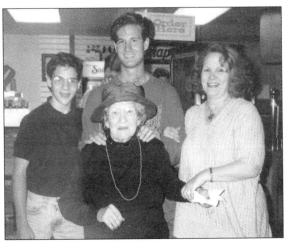

Max, Dirk, Moose and I after Dirk and Brandy's engagement.

recounted the conversation we just had with her grand-parents. Her response was not surprising, considering she had been disowned twice by them, but since had guardedly received them back into her life each time. She stated that if they couldn't share in one of the most impor-tant days of her life and put the differences aside, she would have nothing more to do with them. I can't say that I blamed her, but recognizing this as a potentially explo-sive situation, I tried to diffuse it.

The next day I called my in-laws and tried to explain that we needed to honor both Dirk's Christian heritage and Brandy's Jewish roots. I told them that I would ask the rabbi if he would perform the Jewish part of the cere-mony. We had already procured the Bichsel's pastor to perform the nuptials. They were pleased to hear that we would try to honor them this way. They knew our rabbi because he presided over the reaffirmation of their vows on their 50th wedding anniversary. A peace offering was in the making. We then called the rabbi, who holds himself out to be the bridge between the Jewish and Christian communities and is a good friend of the pastor who would be performing the Christian part of the ceremony. He told us that if it were anyone else, he would've refused imme-diately, but that he would pray about it and get back to us. In the meantime, we plod along making plans.

11/3 For me, it is a bittersweet time preparing Brandy for her wedding, my mother for her death and myself for letting them both go. A little over a week ago, Barry and I spent two nights at a bed and breakfast here in town. It was a gift that the kids had gotten us for our anniversary – which was four and a half months ago. The children and Tammy and Rosie watched Moose so we could break away. I hadn't realized how tense I was until

59

we left the house.

My body suddenly felt as if I had been beaten with a baseball bat. It's amazing how the body tries to compensate while accommodating stress. It was a wonderful time. The kids sprung for the honeymoon cottage, which was decorated so sweetly with comfort in mind. It had a private outdoor jacuzzi overlooking the mountains, fireplace, marble bathroom and a double leather reclining chair facing the television. They even furnished a supply of old movies in the main house, which Barry rummaged through as we checked in. He selected a good variety for our viewing pleasure that night. We went out to dinner at Corbetts (an upscale restaurant), came home, got comfortable, lit a fire and watched our first movie with a comforter over us. It was so intimate and cozy. Afterwards, we went outside for a jacuzzi and watched the moon peaking through the pine trees. We were so relaxed, I felt my body slowly releasing the pent-up tension. We went back inside to watch another movie and fell asleep in the recliner.

11/4 The next morning, we had breakfast in the main house. Much to our surprise, the other guests were also from Colorado Springs. So we shared a gourmet breakfast and good conversation with them. It was a beautiful, crisp, autumn day and the snow storm the weatherman had predicted eluded us. Barry had promised to do a business presentation before we planned this weekend, so he would be leaving our little love nest for a little bit. Until he left, we sat side by side reading the Bible. I was doing a study and he was preparing a sermon to fill in for our pastor the following morning.

I lit another fire and we silently sat next to one another, steeped in the Word. We ate delicious left overs from the previous night's dinner. This private time together was savored like a fine wine until he had to leave. I was content to continue my reading by the fire. It was such a treat to be able to read uninterrupted by the phone, my mother, or the kids. When Barry returned, we watched another movie and planned our dinner.

We decided to go out and collect our favorite foods bringing them back to the cottage for our evening meal. We purchased a special bread and pastries from a wonderful German bakery, and ribs, salad and baked potato from our favorite rib place. We ran back to our haven, settling in for the night. The food never tasted so good. We watched another movie. The next day when we awoke, the storm had come. A white blanket of snow covered everything. We bundled up and went to the main house for another fabulous breakfast. When we returned, there was a call from our daughter saying church had been cancelled and encouraging us to stay there longer, which we did. It was a wonderful time with the Lord and each other. We recognized the need to do this frequently to refresh ourselves spiritually and physically. It was good to rekindle the intimacy and closeness as a husband and wife. Discovering that our libidos were still intact was a relief to both of us.

11/12 *I write when I can. It's nearly impossible finding time to journal when I'm trying to be diligent in two Bible studies, prepare Brandy for marriage, i.e. plan the main event, shop for her trousseau, polish her culinary skills, etc., and give Max the attention he deserves, as well as keeping up on other relationships. I do though, love this time in my life.*

It's nice to be needed. Brandy seems to enjoy long discussions about marriage and is relishing all the benefits deserving of a bride. I'm copying all her favorite recipes to put in a nice book. We are also working on polishing some of the rough edges to make her a more user friendly roommate like not grazing while standing in front of the fridge or eating cold leftovers for breakfast. Max is beginning to explore his manhood asking questions about what girls like. Barry is finding fulfillment in Excel.

Meanwhile, we watch Moose disappear a little each day, desperately trying to hold on to any semblance of normalcy. This is a bittersweet time and one that I'm savoring. Sometimes, I'll be driving in the car and feel overwhelmed with emotion – so happy for my daughter, graduating from college with honors, marrying the man of her dreams. And then, I start to cry because it means she'll be leaving us soon and also, for my mother because she will be leaving too.

Once a week, we get together. Moose, Brandy, the girls and I, work on ceramics projects for Christmas gifts. I make dinner and we sit around painting, talking and noshing (Yiddish for "eating"). It's reminiscent of the old sewing circles where all manners of things are discussed, i.e. weddings, cooking and politics. I wanted Brandy to develop outside interests as next year she'll be living and working with her new husband. We talked about it being crucial that she develop independent interests.

Last week, there were just four of us; Tammy, Rosie, Moose and I. Soon, Brandy joined us. Then, her friend, Mare, stopped by and finally, Max joined in. The only drawback to this wonderful evening of sharing between generations, was that Moose misperceived the people joining in as an attempt by Brandy to push her aside. She spent that night and the next day with an attitude problem. Despite Brandy's attempts to make peace and even apologizing for any perceived wrongdoing, Moose remained aloof. Finally, after Barry sternly chided

Moose by saying, "We don't hold grudges in this household," Moose relented. She responds well to Barry's occasional limit setting for unacceptable behavior.

Fortunately, Moose still has the intelligence to know when to back down. I choose to believe that her behavior is a by-product of the disease. Yet, I know that limits have to be set or she will stay in her delusion. She seems so frail – like when her hands shake as she reaches for something, or her face gets a pained expression, or when she futilely attempts to construct a sentence. Once when we were driving alone in the car, I told her that she was a good mother and had done her best. I don't think she understood. If she did, there was no perceptible response.

I vacillate between feelings of compassion and anger when I can't settle her down. We are having more "bad days" as she is often upset and discombobulated. I'm told that this is the most difficult phase of the disease for her because she is still aware enough to know she is losing her mind. The next anticipated phase, when she won't even recognize family members, is actually easier for her, but is more tragic for the family.

11/20 Today is Moose's birthday. I've ordered a special cake for the senior luncheon at the Temple and tonight, I'm making fillet mignon stuffed with lobster for Tammy, Rosie and Alan. I bought Moose a fur-trimmed hat to match her winter coat and a check to buy more clothes. I try to make these occasions festive and memorable. I know that lately she hasn't exactly been the center of attention with so much else going on and it's hard on her.

11/20 Later – Everyone loved the cake and there was enough left over to serve at dinner. Tammy, Rosie and Alan brought two bottles of Asti Spumante – a lovely

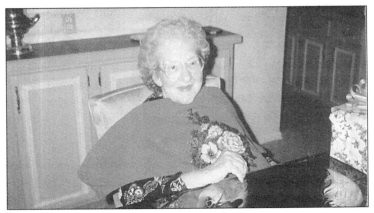

Moose on her birthday.

addition to a good dinner. They made a red jogging suit decorated with poinsettias for the holidays for Moose. She looked great in it. Reuben and Sheryl called twice, but did not even send a card. Todd, my nephew, called as well. I'm glad she doesn't really understand how delinquent they've been, it would be too painful.

11/17 I forgot on the Sunday before Moose's birthday, the girls and Alan had us over for a Mexican dinner. We had a great evening. The food was delicious. That night, however, Moose kept insisting we leave early. I felt manipulated and resentful, wondering when my life would be my own again.

11/27 *Thanksgiving.* We went to the Bichsel's even though Moose has some delusion about Barbara not liking her because Barbara didn't talk to her at a Republican fund raiser event. I told her she would have to go because the girls were going to Texas for the holiday and I wouldn't let her stay alone. Dirk was in Minnesota, but his brothers, Steve and Sterling, were there. Stan did the turkey on the grill, and it was juicy and tender. I brought pecan pie, chocolate whipped cream cake, three breads and a corn souffle. Moose contributed a box of candy and we also sent a floral arrangement. We poured over pictures of Dirk as he was growing up and other family photos. Brandy and I selected some great photos to make into a video for the wedding, composed of each child as they were growing up. The food was delicious and the feeling between the two merging families was warm and joyful as it has been since the beginning. Moose was pretty good, but began to kvetch (Yiddish for "complain") around 7:00 p.m. It had been a long day and she wanted to go home. I tried to get her to take a nap so we could stay longer, but she wasn't having any of it. Once again, I felt manipulated and resentful at having to cut my evening short to accommodate her. I guess I was feeling the effects of how my world had changed since assuming responsibility for Moose. However, she had behaved herself and was fairly social.

11/28 *Friday.* I got tickets for Max, Brandy, Moose, Barbara and I for the Nutcracker Ballet. The sets were magical and costumes beautiful. It was fabulous and Moose was very attentive the entire performance. I asked her if she had ever seen the Nutcracker and she replied that she didn't think so. Exposing her to as much stimulation as possible is a real turn-on for me, especially introducing her to a new experience. I want to take advantage of all that the holiday season offers. It could be her last Thanksgiving, Christmas or birthday and I want it all to be special. We also have tickets for Handel's Messiah and a play – Joseph's Amazing Technicolor Robe. Also, for Brandy's birthday, we are going up to a comedy club in Denver. Tonight, Barb Nelson is coming over and we are having another turkey dinner.

Afterwards, we are going to the tree lighting ceremony at the Broadmoor Hotel, always a festive event.

This morning, Moose came upstairs wearing only her new hat and underpants. She has been constipated, which is usually followed by diarrhea. Getting and keeping her regulated has been a challenge. I found feces in the living room and at this stage, I can't tell if it belongs to my mother or Nibbles, our aging dog, who is in a similar condition.

Moose is having difficulties negotiating the stairs. We placed the house on the market in order to get something with less steps, and it was shown yesterday. I'm tired of cleaning it and getting it ready for showing. We have made an offer on another home on one level. The house has four bedrooms on one level and an apartment downstairs where the girls could live. Our offer was rejected. God seems to be closing doors and I find myself wondering if I will ever have my dream of living on water. We can't seem to find anything, anywhere, that is affordable. I know that the timing for everything is in God's hands. He promised me the desires of my heart if I would be patient and I am standing on that promise. That thought keeps me going.

Delight thyself also in the Lord and He shall give thee the desires of thine heart. Psalm 37:4

Something very dear transpired between Barb and my mother tonight. Barb was expressing concern over one of her children and asking for prayer. My mother walked over to her, placed her hands on Barb's shoulders, looked right at her and said, "Everything is going to be okay." There seemed to be a deep soul-to-soul connection. Anyway, these moments of lucidity coming from Moose now, are startling and welcomed.

12/96 *This holiday season was most memorable and festive. Dirk came in, roses in hand for his mother and me. He is very thoughtful and sweet. We met at Red Robin for lunch and then did some last-minute Christmas shopping. We decorated the house complete with a nativity scene that the girls contributed. Moose hit the ceiling when she saw the nativity scene. We had a long discussion about it, or maybe I should say, argument. We told her this was our belief. We are Jews who accept Christ as our Messiah, but we also honor our Jewish roots and put up a Menorah and celebrate Channukah. The conflict subsided.*

Brandy had two of her friends from Vanderbilt come in to "check out" Dirk. They were perfect guests. They went to sleep late, got up late, helped themselves to breakfast, lunch, or whatever snacks they felt like. Any change in our daily habits knocks my mother for a loop. Having additional people in the house was no exception. Like a two year old resents sharing a parent, Moose let it be known that she didn't like me talking to other people. She began making rude comments to one of Brandy's friends, Julie. I had to correct Moose sternly and apologize to Julie, who was a doll. We planned a big New Year's Eve party for Brandy's friends to meet Dirk. The girls helped me shop and cook, and as long as we were staying in, we invited a few of our friends as well. Dirk and Brandy had a pretty full schedule, making wedding decisions and seeing two different pre-marital counselors.

We kept the girls busy hiking and skiing. The house was full of merriment, with the exception of Moose, who viewed our guests as intruders. My guess is that she likes her world to be small. It must signify safety – knowing what to expect. New Year's Eve, Moose retired early. I felt bad and went downstairs to see if she wanted to toast in the New Year, but she was sound asleep.

Chapter XII

THE FALL

1/97 Things settled down into a comfortable routine after the holiday. We got a contract on our house and things were looking up. We made another offer on the house with the apartment, which was accepted. We were relieved because Moose was wandering around the house more at night, and we were fearful of her falling down the stairs in the dark. Our worst fears came to fruition early on January 11th.

Earlier in the day it was snowing. We had taken Moose over to the new house to pick out the bedroom she wanted for her own. She loved being part of the decision making process. In spite of the upbeat prospect of getting a new house, I had a strange foreboding feeling all day. Moose followed me from room to room, craving attention. I kept trying to allude her to have some alone time. I was all peopled out from the holidays. I remember feeling guilty for wanting to be away from her and thinking I would be sorry later. That evening was a planned women's night out with some friends. Max and Barry took Moose out for dinner.

I really enjoyed the time away. The house was dark and quiet when I returned home that night. Barry was asleep, but I awakened him to ask how his evening went. He said that Moose had been real observant and alert at dinner and that they had a good time, and had no problem putting Moose to bed. Later, she came up to our bedroom and we walked her back downstairs and tucked her into bed. At 1:00 or 1:30 a.m., she got up again and we went through the same drill of walking her back downstairs. I was awakened at 3:30 a.m. to a loud commotion. Barry dashed out of bed and ran downstairs to witness Max trying to lift Moose off the floor onto a chair. They yelled at me to get up. I raced downstairs to face the reality of our worst fear.

Moose had fallen and was in terrible pain. One of us called 911. I rode with her in the ambulance and asked if they could administer something to relieve the pain – it didn't seem to make a dent.

I remember thinking how quiet and deserted the streets were at that time of day. Moose was frightened and so was I. Luckily, the emergency room wasn't crowded due to weather and the early hour. After a series of x-rays, the doctor on call told us Moose had fractured her pelvis in two places. No operation would be needed, only bed rest and physical therapy could heal it.

Moose was admitted into the hospital and we made the decision that one of us needed to be with her around the clock to help avoid confusion and disorientation. Rosie and Tammy agreed to take the 11:00 p.m. to 7:00 a.m. shift so we could go home and rest. They gave my mother strong sedatives and pain killers so she could sleep. She was on oxygen and IV's.

Our main concern was pneumonia setting in, a common occurrence among elderly patients who remain inert for any length of time. Within a very short period of time, we were facing the onset of pneumonia. Friends came and prayed. Food was brought to our home. I was not ready to lose my mother.

An odd thing happened in the hospital. Moose began to talk more lucidly than she had in months. We concluded that the additional oxygen to her brain helped. She actually started reading the commercials on the TV and speaking in full sentences.

The doctor, however, spoke in guarded terms, after all, here was an 82-year-old woman with Alzheimer's, multiple fractures and pneumonia. The prognosis was not good. They treated the pneumonia aggressively with strong antibiotics. I asked God not to take her now. I needed another chance to show him I could care for her without complaining – the usual bargaining that takes place when a loved one is critical. We spoke to Kenny, her conservator, twice daily so he could keep my brother informed of Moose's condition.

In addition to our concern about her physical struggle, we were concerned about Moose's soul. Max was Moose's staunchest prayer warrior. Since her move to Colorado, he prayed for her salvation constantly. He just couldn't comprehend how God would be able to reach an 82-year-old, demented woman. I'd tell him, "He was able to reach you at only age five. God can do anything."

As Moose lay in a critical state, the issue of her salvation was foremost in our thoughts. Moose has been very tolerant of our family's decision to accept Jesus as

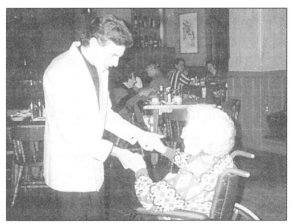

Max with Moose.

our Messiah, eight years earlier. She stated, "I'm too old to argue about religion. If believing in Jesus brings you peace and joy, go for it."

One evening, before the girls arrived for the night shift to relieve us, Moose reached her hand up towards the ceiling and called, "Jesus Christ, Jesus!" Barry and I could tell, the Lord had revealed himself to her. From that moment on, we were all assured of her salvation.

The Holy Spirit was at work in my mother's life and ours as well. I had a strong feeling that we needed to get my mother out of the hospital, where the prevailing attitude was pessimistic. They even stopped feeding her, alleging she could no longer swallow properly. Yet, she ate for us. The Holy Spirit was leading me to bring her home. We went to her doctor, who happened to be a personal friend of ours, and asked for his help in getting whatever services, supplies and medical staff she was entitled to through Medicare and insurance. We were determined. If she was going to die, I wanted her to be at home in familiar surroundings with people who believed in God's healing power.

We were able, with the help of social services, to arrange for home health care including physical therapy, occupational therapy, speech therapy (to help with swallowing techniques), IV setup and a hospital bed with a porta-potty. We got her dismissed and took her home in an ambulance. She had presence of mind to implore us to get her out of there as well. Nurses were sent to our home to teach us how to set up the IV's and change them ourselves. We were barraged with information. I felt like I graduated from a crash course in nursing. The IV's were delivering strong doses of antibiotics and pain killers.

Chapter XIII

CHICKEN SOUP – THE NINTH WONDER OF THE WORLD

That first day back home, I made a double strength pot of chicken soup. I was determined to nurse Moose back to health. She was hooked up to IV's for a week and a half when the tube came out and her veins collapsed. That meant we had to give her enough nourishment orally to sustain her. Also, new medications had to be ordered to be given orally to combat the pneumonia and manage the pain. My mother's physician, our family doctor, friend and neighbor, never once spoke to us or contacted us personally in regards to her medication, care or condition. I was filled with a myriad of emotions, anger, being the strongest, in addition to disappointment, frustration, sadness, etc. I promised myself that we would make her live long enough to switch doctors. My mother responded to the medication, but most of all I believe she responded to all the love and attention we heaped upon her, not to mention the chicken soup!

Slowly, the pneumonia cleared up and the healing process began. She needed less pain medication. Physical therapists came out to teach us how to move her, bathe her, feed her and rehabilitate her. I allowed myself to believe she could make a full recovery and had high hopes of her returning to where she had been before the accident. This, of course, was contrary to the professionals' belief that any catastrophic event could throw an Alzheimer's patient into a new level of deterioration. We elected to believe in God, not what the world's report was. Essentially, we had already beaten the odds. The medical world had us taking her home to die, since according to them she would no longer be able to swallow normally making it impossible to take foods orally. Here we were two weeks out of the hospital and she was alive and eating!

I set small goals for all of us. If she were to get better we had to return to some normalcy. She had to start getting dressed and being brought to the table to eat sitting up. I had consultations with a nutritionist as to how to keep her weight on.

From this time forward, we were always concerned with her nutritional status, trying anything that might help improve her memory, such as ginkgo biloba, niacin and Vitamin E. Each of these were effective, but only for a time. In addition, we experimented with baby foods, pulverized table food, invented high calorie drinks with ice cream, fudge, tofu, protein mixes, etc.

I had the girls give her manicures, cut her hair and put on her make-up. That's what makes me feel human again after an illness. Therapists came to teach us how to get her up walking again. I felt triumphant and she was doing just great although her speech had reverted back to be incoherent after she was taken off of the oxygen.

All the while, Barry was working on our business and had earned a promotion. When I was certain Moose was going to survive, I planned a surprise party for Barry. It was not only a celebration in his honor but also, to give thanks that Moose was still among the living. The first hurdle was figuring out how to get Moose down the front steps and into a car to get to the party.

We decided to do a dry run the week before the party. We had purchased a limo and hired Alan, Rosie's brother, as our driver. The girls came over to get Moose dressed. It was a warm sunny Sunday afternoon in February. Alan pulled the limo over to the sidewalk. I gave Moose enough pain killer to dull any discomfort. We carried her wheelchair down the stairs and managed to maneuver her into the car. She seemed pleased to get out of the house, and as an added treat, we decided to take her to her favorite Vietnamese restaurant where they knew her by name. Gratefully, nobody was there but us. We rolled her in the wheelchair and they made a great fuss over her. We ordered her favorite shrimp dish with egg drop soup.

Moose ate ravenously. I was so touched to see her enjoying food, we ran out and invited Alan to join us for lunch. I realized that eating out was one of Moose's greatest pleasures before the accident, and if we could show her that she could do it again we were on the road to recovery. Our dry run was a success and Alan was so moved he wouldn't accept any money for driving.

The following Sunday, February 16, we carried off, without a hitch, a surprise celebration for Barry – 60 guests at a hotel and Moose was there! Barry and Max's band entertained and people roasted Barry. I was thrilled for him and proud to be able to accomplish two things – arrange a surprise in the midst of all the stress and get my mother back into society. We were on our way back to normalcy, or so I thought.

Chapter XIV

WELCOME TO LALALA LAND

3/97 In early March, my mother waged another battle against pneumonia – not a good sign. I was terribly despondent since March 5th was the anniversary of my dad's death. I prayed I wouldn't lose my mother at this time. The nurses said that we could expect reoccurrences of pneumonia because of Moose's swallowing problems. The head nurse spoke openly in front of my mother, stating that with each onset, my mother's ability to fight back would weaken and that she would never get back to where she was before the accident.

She mentioned Alzheimer's and what the horizon held in store for us. She basically said my mother would at the most, live 6 months to a year longer. To my knowledge, my mother never knew she had Alzheimer's until then when the medical staff talked about it in front of her. I was livid. The nurse suggested we call in Hospice. Reluctantly, I made an appointment, refusing to buy into all the negativity. It was difficult to admit that my mother wouldn't make a complete recovery. I fervently believed we could get my mother walking again.

I was in denial. My mother was exhibiting signs of regressing in the disease. Her muscles began to atrophy and she became more rigid in her hands and legs. Her speech was greatly affected and she developed echolalia, whereby a person repeats a sound constantly. In her case, it was "lalalalalala" all her waking hours. At first, not knowing what it was, I'd try shushing her and became annoyed when she refused to stop. Truthfully, I wanted to slap her, shake her, or do anything to interrupt the constant drone. With much prayer, she made it through her second bout of pneumonia. However, the symptoms she developed lingered on. We did change doctors and kept experimenting with different drugs to give us all some peace.

We had many different nurse's aides come because we realized we needed more help. Rosie and Tammy had their own health issues and Moose's condition was taking a toll on everyone. Some CNA's (certified nurse's aide) lasted only a short time because of the difficulty being around someone who is constantly making noise. It was a sorting process and those who stayed on were worth their weight in gold.

One gentleman, a retired medic from the military, would come from 11 p.m. to 7 a.m. so we could get some sleep. We were all suffering from sleep deprivation. Jerry would arrive like a gentle giant (he's over 6 feet) and stay at Moose's bedside while we got some shut-eye. Jerry brought Moose a t-shirt that said, "I Brake For Moose." It became my favorite article of clothing for her. On Easter, we went to the Bichsel's and Jerry came to stay with Moose. Upon our return, we climbed the stairs and saw Jerry sitting with his arm around Moose on the couch, telling her stories about the Philippines. She was quiet when he told her stories and very attentive. Once he started to tell her the story of *The Three Pigs* and she said, "I've heard that one." She prefers his war stories.

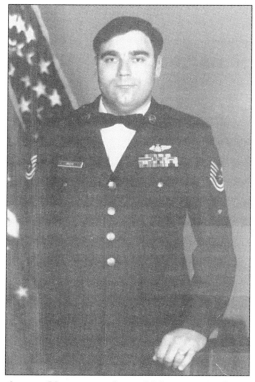

Jerry. Moose preferred his war stories.

We have finally found a medication that lets her sleep through the night, so Jerry only comes as needed now. Moose calls Jerry her boyfriend and likes to have lipstick on when she knows he is coming to be with her.

Another young gal who was a third-year nursing student, came each morning to help get Moose up and dressed. It was difficult for her because Moose became verbally abusive. I held my breath and told her not to take offense – we all got slammed by Moose.

Chapter XV

LIFE GOES ON

4/30/97 It's now nearly May, almost four months after the fall. Moose is alive physically, but is slipping away mentally. Her pleasures are few. She still enjoys riding in the car, the motion lulls her to sleep. Right now, she loves peanut butter sundaes (she only enjoys things for a very short time and then we hunt for something new). She no longer likes to watch television, her attention span is nonexistent. We don't eat with her at the dinner table because we need peace and quiet during meals. We occasionally take her out to eat at the Vietnamese restaurant, where they give her food and don't charge us for it. They love her there and honor us for taking care of her. In my search for finding new places to take her that won't be disturbed by the noises she makes, I discovered the food court at the mall.

We discontinued all therapy for her. She no longer attempts to string beads, paint or do ceramics. She is, for the most part, incontinent and wears diapers all the time now. She is no longer appropriate for the senior program at the temple because of the echolalia. Less and less of what she says, is comprehendable.

In terms of how we are all doing – it's complex. Brandy has other diversions to occupy her thoughts and time. She's a collage senior, graduating with distinction, in spite of all the tumult at home. She's working part-time and we are planning her wedding. These are the bright spots for all of us to focus on. Her first shower is

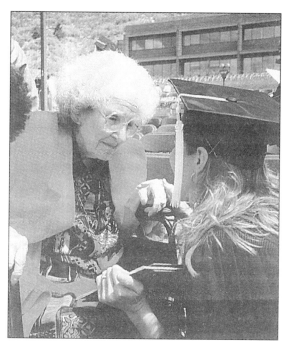

Moose and Brandy at graduation.

the weekend of graduation since her grandparents, aunt and uncle, will be in to celebrate, as well as her fiance. It will be a time of celebration; graduation, shower, Max's 15th birthday and his grandfather's 80th. I wanted so badly for my mother to be with us mentally so she could derive a little pleasure. I know Brandy is affected by Moose's decline, but she keeps so busy – her exposure is less.

Max is a different story. For a 14-year-old, he has had to grapple with a lot of loss in his life. He keeps things bottled up inside and that concerns me. He has fewer outlets and most of his social life is centered around the house.

Barry could be happy in a mud puddle. He's just that kind of guy. This is obviously an emotionally

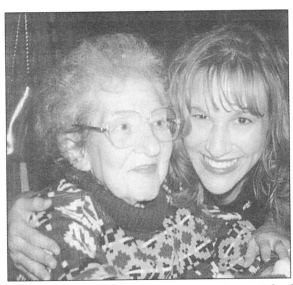

Moose and Brandy at the Vietnamese restaurant for lunch.

charged time for all of us. He's losing a daughter to whom he's always been very close. Physically, it has become very difficult for Barry and Max to carry Moose in her wheelchair, up and down stairs to get her out of the house.

We've begun looking for houses again, as if there isn't enough going on in our lives already. In spite of all this, Barry remains totally upbeat.

As for me, I can't quite keep my emotions in check. I do most of my mourning while driving in the car. It is amazing that I don't get into accidents. God must be watching out for me. I just pray that he allows Moose to be here for the wedding. There is some deep need on my part to have her with me, sharing that time.

5/97 The festivities this month were grand – much better than anticipated. We had a wonderful time with Barry's family. I must admit, I was a bit apprehensive about them meeting Dirk's family. We prepared the Bichsels for the worst possible scenario. Instead, everyone really enjoyed each other. It was such a pleasure. Moose rose to the occasion with not a single "lalalalala" uttered. We celebrated the birthdays by taking everyone, including Moose, out to dinner at the Broadmoor Hotel. We danced, we toasted, we joked. It was delightful. We returned to the house where we had cake and coffee. The birthday cake I made, featured an old model car for my father-in-law, and a sports car for Max. It was the first time we were together to celebrate both birthdays.

Spirits were soaring. Brandy graduated magna cum laude. It was a beautiful day. Janet (Barry's sister), Brandy, Dirk, Jan (a friend of Brandy's), and I rode in the limo to the ceremony. We left early to save seats for everyone. I was busy taking pictures on our new camcorder, memorializing these precious moments.

After the ceremony, Brandy put her graduation cap on Moose. We went to the Vietnamese restaurant for lunch. The food was great. I had a cake brought in. We gifted Brandy with my charm bracelet made into a necklace. I love creating sentimental treasures to be passed on for generations. My grandmother had given this to me and it had charms commemorating events in my life. I had new charms put on for Brandy. Hopefully, she will keep adding charms and pass it on to her daughter.

The following day was Brandy's first bridal shower, given by my friends, Paulette and Betty, at the Antler's Hotel. Brandy and I had our hair done. She looked great and was very charming. My friends did a super job and she received many fabulous gifts.

Dirk, Barry, Michael, Max and George brought

Moose after the lunch, to watch the gifts being opened and to share in the cake afterward. These few days were magical. There was so much love and mutual respect for one another and a shared happiness that was beyond words. I cherish this time.

6/97 Several weeks following the graduation, we met Barry's parents and brother in Palm Springs. We were on a shopping expedition to find a home for us and, possibly, Barry's parents. It was a well needed vacation and, once again, we had a splendid time with Barry's family. We visited one of Moose's long time friends, Edith Levine, who lives with her daughter and son-in-law. I videotaped the reunion to show Moose. It was amazing to see how well Edith was doing at 89 compared to Moose at age 82. We put several offers in on properties, but nothing came of them. From California, we went to see my friend, Nancy, in Las Vegas and were on the same plane with her mother, who lives in Colorado Springs.

When we returned, we sold our home to our friends, the Loewen's. What a surprise! We went back to the original home we had put a contract on and purchased it. So, on top of everything else going on, we are moving to a home more suitable for Moose by summer's end. The new home has an apartment and we spoke to the girls about moving in. Barry is opposed to the idea. He doesn't want his privacy infringed upon, but I can't see not having full-time help. Taking care of the house (over 10,000 square feet), making wedding preparations, caring for Moose, and remodeling the house, would all just be too overwhelming for me.

7/97 Brandy left for Minnesota for two months to

stay with a Christian family who live near Dirk so she would have an opportunity to spend more time with her fiance. I encouraged her to do this as her relationship with Dirk had developed long distance - Brandy in Colorado and Dirk in Minnesota. I'll miss her terribly, but life goes on here.

We began disassembling the house and have boxes everywhere. Moose seems okay with the idea of moving. We keep telling her she will have her own bedroom and bathroom to give her the privacy she's had to do without in this house. I've consulted with various people from the Alzheimer's Association and the Well, an adult program where we take Moose, to get advice on how to make the move an easy transition for Moose. Change can cause a permanent set back to a person suffering from Alzheimer's. We were advised to put Moose in a day program on the day we move, and to get her room set up right away so she won't be too disoriented. I'm told that if she sees anyone taking her possessions, she may get frightened or paranoid. So we talk about the move and all the positive aspects of the new house. Moose had seen the house and had even picked out her room on the day before her fall. She cryptically said, "Buy it." Since there will be no stairs to negotiate when getting her in or out of the house, it will be easier for all of us. It was an answer to prayer and I can't wait to get there.

8/97 Brandy returned a few days before the move, still in love and ready to proceed with the wedding arrangements. There were still two more showers and a dinner party before the main event. We had started making the invitations in June, a project that quickly took on major proportions. Had I known the problems inherent in the project, I would've never done it. But, nevertheless, there was much to be done between the move, the wedding, the remodeling and Moose's well-being. One Saturday evening, we returned home after a movie to hear the tragic news of Princess Diana's death. It was an event that sent shock waves around the globe. Like most people, I was absorbed by the momentous tragedy and loss. The funeral was on moving day. I watched as much as I could, but I had other things on my mind. Moose went to the Well that day and we brought her back to the new house. I am thankful that she never did seem to suffer any set back. After much anguish in our family discussions, "the girls" moved into the apartment downstairs. Anyone who has moved understands the chaos and confusion that accompanies changing residences.

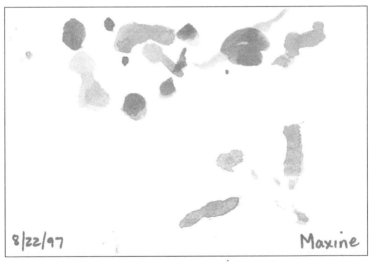

8/22/97   Maxine

Artwork Moose created at the Well.

Chapter XVI

AM I CRAZY?

9/97 We were now seven people under the same roof. Each day contained an endless list of things to do, get, order and make. I'd lay in bed at night and make a mental list of the next day's agenda.

We purchased a baby monitor for Moose's room with the receiver to alternate between the girls' apartment and our bedroom on the weekends. That insured Moose's needs being tended to during the night and we could all get some rest.

The house was bedlam – a constant stream of people coming and going, including wall-paper hangers, tile layers, landscapers, painters, etc., etc., and still endless details and projects to address for the wedding. It was September 6th and the invitations, as protocol dictates, needed to be mailed no later than the 15th. Fortunately, the girls were very artsy craftsy and helped tremendously with various projects.

The chuppa and its construction, brought up another huge project. The chuppa is the canopy under which the ceremony takes place in a traditional Jewish wedding. It represents the new household of the bride and groom. Colorado Springs is not exactly a huge metropolis where you can buy or order anything you want. If I wanted something different for my daughter's wedding, I would have to design it and construct it or hire someone to execute my plan. In this case, I was both the designer and executioner.

I wanted a fairy tale atmosphere for the wedding. The ceremony was to be held at the Fine Arts Center. The room is magnificent but needed to be transformed into a garden-like setting. I rented huge ficus trees to be brought in with twinkle lights to flank either side of the entrance to the room.

Each day I'd foray out to shop for wedding items and decorator items for the house. The countdown had begun. All the while, I felt schizophrenic – a crazy mixture of sadness that I was losing my mother (God willing, she would make it to the wedding), and sadness mixed with elation that Brandy was leaving me too. I'd drive around town like a crazy person, suddenly bursting into tears. I had never had such a frenetic period in my life.

My lifelong dream has always been to plan a detailed, very elaborate and beautiful wedding for my one and only daughter. But, now that the time has come, I somehow have to divide my time and energy between planning the wedding, my daughter and her emotional needs, and the needs of my mother who has become jealous over the time I am spending with Brandy and on the wedding details. When Brandy and I have to run out to do various errands, Moose gets angry and lets everyone know it.

One of the features of our new home was a crafts room which became the wedding center where we pasted, glued and created everything – gift baskets for the out-of-town guests, little gold champagne cups filled with the traditional white Jordan almonds in netting tied with black and gold ribbon, and programs for each table that were replicas of the wedding invitation. Most of all, we gabbed about life, while Moose kept us company.

WILL THE REAL BRIDE PLEASE WEAR WHITE

During this hectic time, Moose became angry with Brandy. It was like sibling rivalry. The spotlight was now on Brandy instead of her. In child-like fashion, Moose let us know that she did not appreciate the competition. The brewing conflict came to a head one Saturday. We had decided to take Moose shopping for the dress she was to wear at the wedding. Barry, Brandy, Max, Moose and I loaded into the car and headed for the nearest mall. The mall was always exciting for Moose because of all the stimulation. She generally sat quietly in her wheelchair as we strolled through the stores.

This would not be the case that fateful Saturday. We were all in a good mood, excited to find Moose's wedding apparel. We were also relieved, with most of the wedding chores behind us and the majority of the renovations to the house complete. We headed for the large department store that housed the most extensive array of cocktail dresses. Brandy and I perused the racks of lovely frocks, while Max and Barry strolled beside us with Moose. It had been decided that the bride's side of the family would be in black and the groom's family would be in cream.

As we selected several lovely gowns to show Moose, a frown developed on her face. She wanted to wear white. The more we tried to explain that only the bride would be wearing white that day, the more insistent she became. Our voices, out of frustration, went up a decibel or two, until one of us suggested we go home and try this again another time. I said, "Why don't we go to the food court and calmly discuss this over a coke?" So we took time out and all cooled off. We were able to analyze what was taking place. Moose was suddenly able to express herself. She stated, "I have a man too."

I replied, "You can get married another time, it's Brandy's turn. When it's your turn to be the bride, you can wear white." This seemed to appease her enough so we could resume our search. Within 15 minutes, with Moose's approval, we had chosen a pair of black chiffon designer pants with a gorgeous heavily-beaded black top. Everyone was pleased to have accomplished the goal, given the unforeseen roadblocks we had to get around. On the drive home, we all got a chuckle out of the episode. But, it served as a poignant reminder of where Moose was emotionally. I had become the mother arbitrating between squabbling siblings.

Max was not exempt from Moose's outbursts either. Their conflicts centered around toileting procedures. Moose was not totally incontinent. The trick was to catch her before she had an accident. Once we mastered the timing, a routine fell into place. Like clockwork, after dinner, we'd inquire if she needed to go to the bathroom. Invariably, she'd say, "Yes," and the drill would begin. Max, Moose and I would retreat to Moose's room where we'd pull out the porta-potty. Max was responsible for transferring her from the wheelchair to the potty, while I pulled down her outer garments and diaper. Moose would lash out at Max in frustration, digging her nails in and saying, "You, you, you," unable to complete her thought. Max would get irritated and say, "Grandma, stop it. I'm only trying to help."

Then she'd mutter something else and it would escalate until I'd have to intervene with, "Max, just leave the room. Walk away. I'll call you when I need you." Countless times I'd have to remind him that his efforts to explain things to her were futile and that he should ignore her tantrums.

His reply was usually the same, "It's easy for you to say, you're not the object of her anger." His point was well taken. Very rarely did she unleash her anger toward me. Actually, I found these out-bursts hilarious; to see an 83-year-old woman engaged in a fight with a 15-year-old boy, was like watching two siblings go at it.

When I look at it from Moose's perspective (adolescent behavior from a senior citizen), she was probably humiliated at having to depend on others for anything, let alone the very private function of eliminating body waste in such a public manner. She had no privacy anymore. I knew every inch of her body, much to her chagrin, I'm sure. I can only imagine how awful it must have been to have people wiping her behind and cleaning her genitals. After all, as much as we tried to preserve her dignity, she was nevertheless deprived of her privacy. Barry and I discussed on a number of occasions how surprised we were that we were not "put off" tending to Moose's toileting needs. It was as if God had equipped us with skills to rise above the normal response to perform such difficult tasks. It became mechanical. We did what had to be done. There were days that bowel movements lasted an hour in order to relieve her of discomfort. Many times, I'd have to put on rubber gloves and pull out the feces because she had lost muscle tone; an intimate procedure nobody envisions having to do to others or, heaven forbid, having someone do to you. That's what this disease is about – being reduced to the lowest common denominator in terms of human functions. Without belaboring the point, there were days we'd change my mother's diaper 2-4 times, only to discover there was more changing to do.

My mother got the best care and died without one bedsore or skin tear on her body, a feat few caregivers achieve with their patients. All the caretakers we brought in to do shift work would comment on the great condition of Moose's skin.

Before going anywhere we'd check her pants. I was devastated when Moose would remind me, "I'm not a baby." I would answer, "I know, Moose, we just need to make sure you're okay before we leave." The issue of anger, revolving around her toileting procedures, would later be discussed at a family counselling session. At any rate, Moose would have her grudge matches that endured until the end. She was forever angry with Brandy for "stealing her man" and taking my attention away from her.

As I would be going out the door, she'd shoot me a look as if to say, "What about me?" This was reminiscent of when the children were toddlers and would cry pathetically as my husband and I left for the evening. As much as her pleading look tugged at my heartstrings, I knew having "alone time" was essential to preserve my own sanity and health. I would promise Moose that we'd go for a ride or to lunch later. That would satisfy her and give her something to look forward to. How could I explain to her that I only had one daughter who was getting married, and that this was a once-in-a-lifetime experience?

There was so much to be done, i.e., preparing a cookbook with all my favorite recipes for Brandy, trying different hair stylists and hairdos, fittings for dresses, and registering for gifts at department stores. We had so much to do and time was short. Barry, Brandy and I would get up at the crack of dawn to hike to have undisturbed time together. These were precious moments.

Invitations went out in great style. Barry dressed in a tuxedo and we drove in the limo to hand deliver them in town. We wanted every aspect to be special. I had fixed hors d'oeuvres and stocked the limo with soft drinks. We invited Barbara, Dirk's mother, to join us. Again, I observed how bittersweet my life was. My prayer each morning was for strength and that Moose would make it to the wedding.

The fall of '97 was spectacular. We'd take Moose out for walks, the fresh air and scenery seemed to quiet her down. The girls, Tammy and Rosie, were working out fine. We settled into a comfortable routine with them getting Moose up, dressed, and fed each weekday. Afterwards, they would help by doing light house work. I'd hoped that by having hired two people the burden would be shared, lessening the chance for burnout. Ultimately, I would be proven wrong.

The days marched on and wedding responses poured in. Each afternoon we'd race to the mailbox to see who would be attending. The excitement mounted. A week before the wedding, Dirk arrived just as one of the worst snow storms in years hit Colorado Springs. We were snowed in together for three days. My biggest concern was having enough supplies, particularly diapers, for Moose to carry us through. On the fourth day, we managed to dig ourselves out and immediately headed to the nearest grocery store.

I pondered over what the logistics would be like if the weather persisted. We had guests flying in from Hong Kong, New York, Dallas, California and Seattle and inclement weather could be the monkey wrench in everyone's safe and timely arrival. In addition, we had singers and musicians flying in from Oklahoma. We still had a prayer brunch, given by my friend, for our immediate families and two dinners given for the out-of-town guests.

As the Lord commands, *"Be anxious about nothing."* I had to trust that our prayers would cover the situation. The weather cleared up, snow melted and guests arrived as scheduled. All of our careful planning was coming to fruition. Gratefully, Moose was still with us, and understood to some degree what all the tumult was about.

One of my oldest and dearest friends, Pam, arrived early to help, along with one of Moose's favorite people, Michael, my brother-in-law from Hong Kong. Both would be staying with us at the house. The festivities had begun, and, with the arrival of each person, the level of excitement increased. Moose was reluctant to share her space and promptly said to Pam, "Go home." I was a little embarrassed but then thought, "Oh well, this is my world, welcome to it."

Even with Michael, Moose was guarded and told Tammy and Rosie, "Watch out for him. Keep your door locked," referring to his reputation as a ladies' man.

I was torn as my desire for Moose to attend as many of the wedding events as possible, but selfishly, I wanted to be able to enjoy them completely without having to worry about her. I had talked about this for the last year, trying to give her something positive to look forward to. I compromised and she attended the rehearsal (so she would know what to expect at the wedding) and one of the dinners for the out-of-town guests.

My brother-in-law and I have had our "go-arounds" with one another in the past, and in spite of trying very hard to have things go smoothly, we got into it over his smoking. He moved into a hotel in a huff, and that night, at dinner, things erupted again. Moose was sitting beside me and, bless her heart, that motherly instinct to protect her child had not died off; as Michael was getting into a heated discussion with me, Moose raised her finger and shook it in his direction, glaring at him, as if to say, "You leave her alone." That incident evoked powerful feelings in me as I realized that my best advocate was still here to defend me. Everyone needs

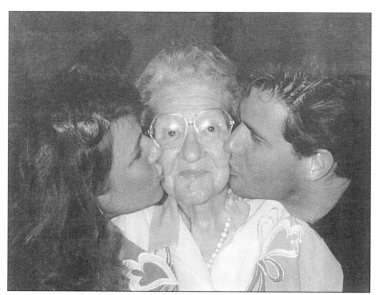

Brandy, Moose and Dirk at the rehearsal dinner.

93

that kind of loyalty and unconditional love in their lives. I think this quality is what I miss most about my mother. Children and husbands, although they love you, have a different kind of love – each powerful, but not the same.

Once, Barry and I were going up to Denver for a Christmas party during questionable weather, the girls told us that Moose wanted desperately to stay up until we arrived home safely. She still had the capacity to worry about me. Sometimes, when I was dressing to go out for the evening, I would go into her room for approval, and she would reach out to pick off a piece of lint from my clothing: a small gesture, but one filled with meaning to me. She was still, and always would be, my mother.

Moose never demonstrated much affection towards me. As a child, I would have to ask for a good-night kiss from her. In the last three years of her life, our roles had certainly reversed to the point of her calling me "Mother." However, those rare moments when she showed maternal instincts stand out like a single red rose in a field of sunflowers. Small, tiny moments left of her career as a mother, yet, they were monumental to me.

The day of the wedding had finally arrived. We hired the male nurse, Jerry (being one of Moose's favorites), to attend to all my mother's needs as each of us readied ourselves for the nuptials. Brandy and I managed to steal away for several hours in the a.m. to get our make-up professionally applied, leaving the others to fend for themselves. Based on my own experience, I advised her to try to soak it all in – there would never be another day like this one in her life. I told her to pause as she stood at the head of the aisle, to recognize that she would be surrounded by love. Everyone there would be single minded in their joy for her and Dirk. Our time together that morning was a treasure I will savor for a lifetime.

That day was as close to perfection as life ever gets. To witness my child lovingly make a covenant before God and her chosen partner was awesome. Moose rose to the occasion looking radiant and – there were no lalalalalala's that day.

I was so proud when my handsome son, Max, escorted Moose down the aisle. She demurely had her hands folded and looked like the Queen Mother. Just as

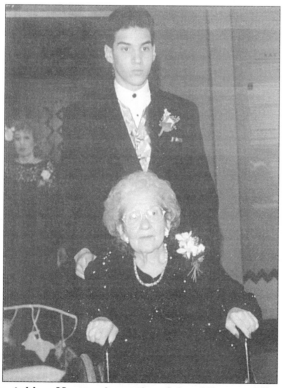

Max taking Moose down the aisle at the wedding.

she approached Dirk, standing alone, waiting for his bride, she reached out her hand to touch his and smiled. There was not a dry eye in the place. It was a poignant moment that passed between the two. As a friend succinctly put it, the day was like a fine wine that continued to be poured out.

All of the frustrations that go along with planning a once-in-a-lifetime event were worthwhile when I saw pictures of my daughter's feet, not touching the ground, as she danced with her new husband. My husband and I had succeeded at crafting a perfect day for our loved ones. God had certainly answered all of our prayers.

For this reason I am telling you, whatever you ask for in prayer, believe that it is granted to you, and it will be yours. Mark 11:24

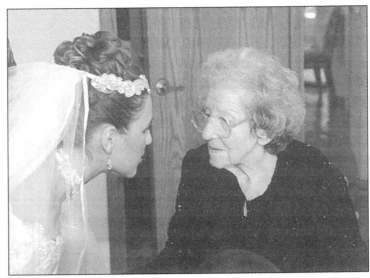

Moose had a hard time accepting all the attention given to Brandy. Moose also wanted to wear white.

The following day, we had a catered brunch at our home for 30 of the out-of-town guests. The girls got Moose up, dressed and tended to her needs, freeing me to play hostess. Moose loved all of the action. However, as we waved good-bye to the last of our guests and kicked off our shoes, there was a sense of relief; I knew that my focus could now be fully directed toward Moose. I no longer had to feel pulled in several directions simultaneously. It was Moose's turn to be the bride. I was thankful to the Lord for allowing Moose to see one of her grandchildren get married. We had reached one of our milestones. For weeks and months afterward, people were telling us what a grand occasion the wedding was.

Chapter XVIII

AROUND THE NEXT BEND

11/97 With the main event over. I could now get back to normal. We had Thanksgiving around the corner, and Moose's birthday to look forward to. I wanted to make a big deal out of Moose's birthday, never knowing if this was to be her last. I got up early that day and baked one of my favorite chocolate cakes from scratch for her. We had made reservations at a new restaurant in town, featuring fresh crab, one of Moose's favorite foods. We invited Tammy, Rosie and Alan, who had agreed to drive us all in the limo.

Bouquets of roses began to arrive. Reuben and Sheryl sent her yellow, long-stemmed roses and we sent red roses. I made a big fuss as each arrived, bringing them to her room and talking about how much she was loved. It was important for me to let her know, in a hundred small ways, how much she meant to us. Like a small child, she kept asking when we were going to the restaurant. Her impatience was showing by 5:30 p.m. and she was in a snit. Adding to Moose's discontent, the restaurant refused to take reservations and we had to wait in line. By the time our food arrived, her black mood eclipsed our attempt to create a celebrative atmosphere. She refused to eat, so I decided to ignore it and had her dinner boxed up to take home.

After dinner, we went back to the house to have cake and coffee. Now she was directing her anger at Alan for no apparent reason. She was rude to him and I had to reprimand her. We tried taking her attention off him by opening presents, but once she got a bee in her bonnet, it was difficult to redirect her attention. I knew I had to stop trying to control her environment. Despite my efforts to create a nice memory for her, other elements would come into play. We may have reached another plateau in terms of restaurant behavior. She used to love to share food with me, but, maybe that phase was over. From that evening on we were limited to where we could take her to eat because her etiquette was vanishing. This event was less perfect than the wedding. I had to confess that I was not capable of creating perfect days for my mother.

Thanksgiving proved to be another disaster for Moose. We had invited the Bichsels, the girls and Alan. It was our first holiday since the kids got married and we were all still on cloud nine. In fact, for weeks and months following the wedding, people would comment on how lovely it was. Anyway, Thanksgiving morning, as Tammy and Rosie were getting Moose dressed, she began fussing. I was up to my eyeballs in work and didn't have time or patience for a temper tantrum. I marched into Moose's room and unleashed on her. I basically told her that she had a lot to be thankful for; she has a loving son-in-law who welcomed her into his home and a family that adores her and wants to take care of her. If she was so unhappy, we could arrange to put her in a home. I told her if she didn't behave today, she could spend time in her bedroom by herself.

She was quiet the rest of the day. Afterward, I felt horrible for unloading on her like that. I was convinced that she couldn't help herself, and did not want to be a burden on anyone. However, her child-like behavior sometimes called for discipline, as much as I hated to administer it. The day went on without incident, but I wondered if somewhere in the recesses of her mind, she had made a decision to let go. She was a fighter, but in looking back, there was a difference from that day forward. My prayer is that I did not say something inadvertently that day to hurt her. I'll never really know because she could never express it to me. How could I have known that this was to be her last Thanksgiving?

Shortly after the wedding, Barry asked me if I'd like to accompany him and a business associate to Washington for some speaking engagements. Feeling a need to wind down and indulge myself, I gladly consented. I wanted to say yes to him more often. He deserved it. There aren't too many son-in-laws who would love their mother-in-law like he did. Besides, I had never been to Washington and it was on my list of places to see. Although the weather was rainy and cold, I had a great time sleeping in late and not worrying about Moose (since we would only be away for a long weekend). As usual, however, I made several calls a day home to check on Max and Moose. We returned home to find that the house had been under siege by a shady character, seen lurking in the field beside our driveway. He had apparently approached the house several times and the girls called the police. Although nothing ever came of it, I was temporarily in a panic mode.

12/97 It was becoming apparent to us that Moose's sister, Lucille, in McAllen, Texas was gravely depressed. A recent widow, with no children, she had nobody to turn to for help. After our return Washington, we booked a flight to Texas in early

December to assess the situation. We had a large home and staff in place – to take in one more family member wouldn't be such a big deal. We thought it would be a boost to both sisters if they could spend their remaining years together. We arrived to find Lucille surprisingly spry, lucid and handling day-to-day living rather well, with one exception; she was having difficulty with her neighbors and the police were being called almost daily. After a week of observing the situation, we convinced Lucille that her best option would be to sell her home and come live with us. She agreed to get her affairs in order and then we'd return to help her move. She had a laundry list of things to be done before marketing her home, although it appeared to be in excellent condition to us. This was going to be a huge step for her and she had to go at her own pace. When we parted company, I believe she had hope for a new life. We had laid the foundation and set her feet on a path. The rest was up to her.

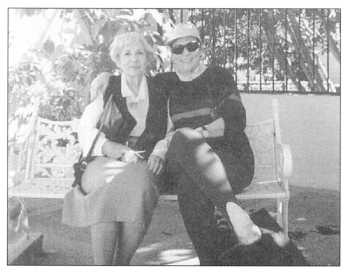

Lucille and I on a daytrip to Mexico.

We arrived back in Colorado to find our home completely decorated for Christmas. The tree was up, the exterior was outlined in red lights and visual delights were in every direction. The girls had been like little elves preparing for our homecoming. I wanted this Christmas to be special. The newlyweds would be returning for the holidays. It would be fun observing our daughter in her new role as wife. I set up a guest bedroom as my gift-wrapping headquarters.

One afternoon, we were making rounds delivering gifts to friends, when suddenly Moose couldn't hold herself upright in her wheelchair. Her head was thrown back and she had marked difficulty breathing. We pulled into a friend's driveway, rushed inside and asked for prayer. It happened to be our pastor's home, and the pastor's wife, Tresa, had lost her mother to Alzheimer's seven months prior. They ran out to the car and begged us to call Hospice, as it looked like Moose was dying. They told us Hospice had helped them through the dying process with Tresa's mother. They dialed the number for us. I didn't want to admit that this could be it. Ron Coffin, the head of Hospice made an appointment to come out and talk with us. In the meantime, we rushed to get Moose home and get her comfortable. We had pre-determined she would die at home – no emergency rooms or hospitals. Home was the last frontier.

Having been down this road before, I asked Barry to phone in a prescription for a potent liquid antibiotic to stave off pneumonia. We managed to get a couple doses down her. As before, her body responded quickly to the medication. Nevertheless, I realized it was time to call in Hospice. That Monday, a representative came out and took the vital information and had me sign the necessary papers. When the girls came up to report for work, having had the weekend off, I brought them up to speed on Moose's condition and the need for calling Hospice. Tammy, the more reactionary of the two, objected, saying Moose wasn't anywhere near ready for that. I described the episode we'd experienced the day before, and explained we needed to face the eventuality of her death. If this was premature, time would tell.

After the interview, the Hospice staff was put into place and the doors to our home were thrown open to welcome them. Three days a week a beam of sunshine named Maria would come to bathe my mother, dress and feed her breakfast. This meant the girls could start their day later giving them an opportunity to sleep in.

Twice a week, a nurse named Peggy, would stop in to take my mother's vital signs, discuss any medical problems we encountered and, if needed, phone the doctor to order the appropriate medication. In addition, I was assigned volunteers for a few hours on Saturday and Sunday, to relieve us on the weekends. Suddenly, there was a flurry of activity in our household with Moose at the center. She was soaking up all of the attention as we adjusted to the schedules and new personalities coming into our home. It was like the changing of the guard.

The hospice staff were like hand-picked angels sent from above to escort us all through the valley of the shadow of death with Moose. Barry, Max and I didn't have to shoulder this tremendous burden alone anymore. At first, I think the girls felt that their job had been taken away – their authority usurped, but soon we all settled into this new phase of Moose's care and like well-greased wheels of a machine, we worked together with the singular purpose of Moose's well-being.

We also had at our disposal the services of a social worker, Rita, to address issues surrounding Moose's care. At first, I didn't see any need for her services. I began to think that we all were in denial and hiding our feelings. Since Dirk and Brandy were coming for the holidays, I thought it would be a great idea to have a family "rap session" – a venue to vent any and all feelings attached to Moose's care. Surprisingly, the kids both said, "We don't need a social worker. We are a very vocal family and can discuss issues amongst ourselves." After all, their father is a shrink. Still, I pressed on with the notion that just beneath the surface, if lightly scratched, there was a host of resentments, anger and sadness to be dealt with. I called Rita and asked if she would be available for my family during the holidays. She readily agreed to facilitate a session for us and a date was set. I never expected my suggestion to meet with such resistance, least of all from my two savvy kids. After all, we were all used to expressing ourselves. Why was this so objectionable to them? I knew I had struck a nerve. The more resistance, the more insistence on my part. Truthfully, it might have been more for me to face my own fears. We had been planning a family vacation for spring break in March and I was reluctant to commit, especially if Moose was in poor health. I was very tentative with my "yes." I couldn't very well go, in good conscience, leaving Moose in ailing health.

Brandy and Dirk arrived from Minnesota, where they were now living, on Brandy's birthday, December 21st. We went out for dinner with Dirk's folks, leaving Moose at home with "the girls." She was still recovering from her episode. I felt terribly guilty and couldn't wait to get home to see Moose. Everyone came back to the house to view the wedding video and see Moose. She was up waiting for us.

By the look on her face, we surmised that Moose didn't recognize Dirk and Brandy. After all, Brandy had been absent from my mother's life for over a month. Perhaps this was another indication that the disease was progressing. However, that glimmer of recognition returned after being with them for the evening.

Watching the wedding video was like reliving the event. We were all awed by the beauty and splendor of that day. The following week we invited the guests who were unable to attend the wedding, to see the video and have a piece of wedding cake I had frozen. I wanted to keep that precious memory alive. We were all basking in the afterglow. That evening, the kids went back to sleep at Dirk's parents' home. How odd to have our daughter in town and not with us; one of the new adjustments we'd all have to make. Life was ever changing and we had to keep rolling with the punches. Brandy was married and we had to share her with another family now. It gave me great pleasure to see how happy they were and how well adjusted to married life they had become in just over a month's time.

As the date for our family session with Rita approached, objections were raised by various participants. I let everyone know that it was totally their choice as to whether or not they attended. It was not mandatory or a punishment, but merely an opportunity to surface feelings. As it turned out, everyone, including Moose and Dirk, decided to come, although Moose snoozed through the entire session.

Brandy was the first to open up. She eloquently

spoke of her regret that Moose openly showed disdain toward her. Rita responded that the disease sometimes causes the patient to lash out at the unexpected, thinking that they are someone else, perhaps someone from their past who had mistreated them. Brandy said that it was difficult being the target of this kind of anger. Then Max spoke up. Until now, he had been slouched in a chair with one leg thrown over the arm. He started, "How do you think I feel when I pick her up to put her on the toilet and she scratches me and tries to hurt me? I hate that. I sometimes want to smack her. But, I know I can't."

Rita responded, "Imagine how frightened Moose must be when, without warning, she's picked up, her pants pulled down and she's transferred to the toilet. She has to rely on everyone to do things for her. It's frustrating as well. Do you think, Max, before you lift her you could let her know what you're going to do and why?"

Max asked, "What do you mean?"

"Well, for example, you could say, Moose, I'm going to have to lift you up now so we can put you on the toilet. Let her know what is going to happen," suggested Rita.

Max stated, "Yeah, I could do that, I guess."

I sat there, mostly listening, glad to see my kids opening up and sharing their darkest feelings toward the situation, but more pointedly, toward Moose. Then Brandy turned the discussion to concerns about me not showing any emotion. I confessed to being a private person who had cried an ocean of tears while driving in my car. That was how I handled my grief – quietly, alone. I had grieved with each ability that Moose lost; I just was not given to public displays of emotion. Rita interjected that I'd probably already done the majority of grieving over Moose and that when she actually passed on, I will be well on my way to healing. I said that I hoped that would be the case, although losing my mother was like losing my best advocate, no matter how incapacitated she was – she is still my mom.

Then Barry asked, "How do you feel about taking a vacation?" I expressed my conflicting feelings about wanting to be with the family, but, that I was afraid to leave Moose, knowing that she views me as her lifeline. How would I feel if she died while I was gone or if she were gravely ill before we left? Rita said this is a common scenario with Hospice patients and their families. Hospice encourages people to go on their vacations, but only after saying everything they need to say to the patient to bring closure in the event their loved one dies while they are gone. She also cautioned me not to put my life on hold while waiting for Moose to die. She assured me that Moose would not want that for me. Everyone chimed in and stated that they needed me too. Their point was valid, so I agreed to go on the vacation in March.

Part of my hesitancy, was because I had committed myself to be with Moose until the end. There is some comfort in knowing that we may have some say as to when we breathe our last breath. Rita related stories to me about other patients who either waited for that last relative to arrive before dying, or waited until everyone left their bedside so they could die alone.

I left the session resolved to say everything I wanted to say to Moose before we took the trip. Not wanting to let a long time lapse from when the suggestion was made, I chose a quiet afternoon to vent my feelings toward Moose. She was sleeping. I rolled her wheelchair into the gift-wrapping room. I started telling her how angry and resentful I was that she always opted to live near Reuben and his family. Reuben, who disrespected her, didn't watch out for her or take care of her, but was her favorite. My family, who begged her to come live with us, were second choice and were left the task of taking care of the shell of the woman she had become. My kids needed her as much as Reuben's and we were the ones who treated her the best. There, I had said it. Moose was still asleep, but I said what was in my heart. Who knows what she may have heard or understood? It didn't really matter. I'd completed my mission. If she died a second later, nothing would've been left unsaid. I'm convinced that's what made my father's death so easy for me to handle. I'd seen him 10 days prior to his death and told him how much I loved him and what a great father he was. There were no regrets – no wishing I had 10 minutes more with him to say that last thing. It was all finished between us and now, it was finished with my mother too. I said, "Okay, God, I'm ready to let go of Moose." Future events would prove me wrong.

The holidays were a festive time. Christmas Eve we dined with Dirk's parents and attended a candlelight ceremony at First Presbyterian. Our small family had doubled in size. We were united through marriage and now shared our holidays with the Bichsels. After the service, we came back to our house to open presents. Moose had stayed awake and there was a blazing fire in the fireplace. We plowed through our gifts as did Moose. Tammy and Rosie were leaving the following day for Texas. Rosie had become a grandmother. I was overjoyed for her as someday myself I looked forward to holding the title of grandmother.

Chapter XIX

EXIT: THE GIRLS

12/97 The girls' departure for Texas for four days left Barry and I as primary 24-hour caregivers. Thankfully, Hospice volunteers would fill in during their absence. We also called a temporary home health care service, who dispatched a young woman to our home. We'd be needing her four days in a row for several hours each day. The first few days, we would be present – we were hosting several parties at home. Those first days enabled her to learn the routine with Moose, while I supervised. She was competent and quite engaging. However, there were a mysterious series of events to come that would be unsettling and have far-reaching ramifications.

On the third day, we decided to go to the movies leaving Moose alone with this aide for a few hours. When we returned that evening, all the lights were turned on in the house and the front door was ajar. The hair on the back of my neck stood up. Something had to be wrong. We ran to my mother's room and there they were watching television. I asked, "Is everything okay?" She said, "Yes, everything is fine, why?" I told her that the front door was wide open. She said she thought there was a rush of cold air, but didn't bother to investigate. We searched the house to see if anything was amiss. She further stated that she'd heard a noise earlier that sounded like we'd arrived home. Satisfied that all appeared okay, we dismissed her for the evening. As we prepared Moose for bed, I looked up to discover the electric eye for the motion detector in Moose's bedroom was dismantled. It was dangling as if someone purposely took it apart. If only Moose could talk! Questions rang in my head. Had the girl left Moose alone and in her haste to return left the door open? Had she invited friends over? Had she spied the electric eye and, thinking it was surveillance, dismantled it so she could go to sleep? The next day, I reported it to the agency, in case we found anything was missing, and to inquire if they had received complaints from other clients about this girl. Thinking it odd, they sent a representative over to investigate. We have since returned the electric eye. It has never fallen again, nor had it before this incident, which leads me to believe this gal, thinking it was a camera, took it apart.

Something happened that night that would shape future events. We were trusting, perhaps too much so, and Moose was unable to defend herself. From that time on I was convinced we needed to set up some kind of surveillance to determine if Moose was being mistreated in our absence. You can't be too careful when the well-being of a defenseless loved one is at stake. I began to make queries of detective agencies as to the cost of setting up hidden cameras. I was quoted prices up to $10,000.00 – an exorbitant amount of money. The whole thrust of this was trying to assure myself that Moose was well cared for in our absence. In a few months, we would all be going away and for the first time, and Moose would be left alone without benefit of a family member present to protect her. I had to know if the girls were totally trustworthy. I nursed this idea for weeks.

2/98 Finally, in February, on Valentine's Day,

Barry and I were going to spend an evening at a hotel and Max would be at a friend's house overnight. This was a perfect opportunity to set the snare. I excitedly went to the local Radio Shack and purchased an inexpensive, voice-activated tape recorder. Planting the recorder under my mother's nightstand, we said our good-byes and headed out the door for our romantic interlude. Then, of course, my paranoia set in. What happens if they find the recorder? I dismissed the thought. Before dawn the next morning, we rushed home to retrieve the recorder. It was right where I left it. I retreated to our bathroom to play back the tape. Much to my relief, I had captured a very nice interchange between Moose and the girls as they prepared her for bed. They asked Moose who had sent her such beautiful flowers for Valentine's Day and told her that they surely must love her because the flowers were so pretty. A sense of well-being flooded over me. Thank God they were good to her. My trust in them was well placed.

Days went by and our vacation was a month away. Something told me to run the tape again, but this time, in a different location. I chose a day when I would be in and out of the house running errands. Carefully, I placed the recorder behind some cookbooks in the kitchen and forgot all about it. Barry was called away on business, so I invited the girls to join Moose, Max and I for dinner. There was a reluctance on their part to accept the invitation. Something wasn't quite right, but I couldn't put my finger on it. They came upstairs and things seemed pleasant enough. In fact, we shared some funny "Moose stories." After dinner, as usual, they got Moose ready for bed. Meanwhile I soaked in a hot bath and Max retreated to his room to do homework.

Remembering the tape, I ran to retrieve it. What unfolded on that tape was horrifying. That simple $50.00 gizmo captured an entire interaction between the girls and my mother. I could hardly believe my ears. What began as the usual frustration in feeding Moose, erupted into a full-scale verbally, mentally and physically abusive scenario that lasted 10-15 minutes. I listened, not wanting to believe what I was hearing. I felt betrayed. There was no turning back or pretending it didn't happen. Action had to be taken. I anxiously awaited Barry's return and presented him with the evidence. It was all I could do to restrain him. He was so enraged he wanted to go down to their apartment and evict them immediately. I cautioned him that this had to be handled carefully. We had to solicit opinions of people in authority. We called our pastor, Chuck, and the head of Hospice, Ron. They both agreed to come early the next morning, listen to the tape and render an opinion on how we should proceed.

The following day was Friday, the girls' late day, which meant they wouldn't be up for work until 11:30 a.m. Chuck and Ron promptly arrived and listened to the tape, independent of one another. Ron spoke first saying that this was abuse on several levels and now that he was aware of it, we had no recourse, but to fire them or he would have to report us to the authorities for placing Moose in a precarious position. I was sick to my stomach. All at once, our lives were turned upside down. You read about these things happening to other people but you don't expect it to happen in your safe haven. At once, my heart went out to poor defenseless Moose. I was so sorry she had been subjected to their tirade and mistreatment, even if only for 10 minutes. However, who knows if this was just an isolated incident. It could have been going on a long time. We discussed giving them a chance to confess which would've suggested some conscience. I called them on the intercom and asked them to come upstairs. They had been exercising in the gym. Ron opened the discussion by asking how they were doing, with respect to the job of caring for Moose. They, not knowing what was going on, maintaining a casual air, said everything was fine. Ron said, "Are you certain you girls aren't having any difficulty?" They glanced at one another and shook their heads "no." Ron continued, saying he and Chuck were called to the house because we are all concerned for Moose's welfare and dedicated to providing her with the best care.

The girls nodded in accord. He stated that we had called them because we suspected abuse. They looked at one another with their mouths agape. With their eyes wide like innocent babes they said, "You don't think we've done anything to Moose, do you?"

Barry nearly jumped out of his seat. Pointing a finger toward them, he said, "We have it on tape – the entire interaction yesterday with you screaming at Moose and threatening to 'beat the hell out of her' and calling her stupid and an animal and then apologizing for hitting her."

Tammy's eyes welled up with tears, "Well, Barry, it was a very bad day yesterday and I admit I lost it – but so have we all at times."

Barry, his face reddened with rage, shot back, "It was a bad day for Moose. I wouldn't talk to a dog the way you spoke to her. How long would you work for me if I spoke to you that way? I want you out of here today."

Rosie, her head hanging, said, "So all the good

things we've done don't matter. We lose it once, and we're out of here."

Ron responded, "Even one offense is punishable by law."

Sobbing, Tammy said, "Please, Barry, I'll go for counselling to work on my anger."

I spoke for the first time saying, "Our trust in you has been violated. We can never take the chance of leaving Moose in your care again. You hit her."

Rosie retorted, "Yes, but it was only with paper towels." To which Barry responded, "What next time, a sledge hammer or whatever is handy?"

Ron interrupted, "The Krafts have no choice. As head of Hospice, I'd report them if they didn't take immediate action by dismissing you. I'd have to report the incident to social services, who would remove Moose from the home."

Tammy said, "Please, Barry don't kick us out. This is our home, we have nowhere to go. You've all lost your tempers with Moose."

I answered, "The difference is we've never called Moose degrading names or struck her or threatened to beat her. You are the paid professionals. Rosie, I hold you equally responsible for not interceding on Moose's behalf to protect her. That's why we hired two of you, to spell one another when things get too tough. You did nothing to defend Moose and, in fact, you both ganged up on an 83-year-old, defenseless woman."

Rosie got up and headed for the door saying, "Come on, Tammy, we have to go."

I said, "Rosie, let Tammy speak. I want to hear what she has to say."

Tammy continued to plead her case, saying she

would do anything to keep her job. I retorted, "I would've understood and continued to trust you if you had come to one of us and said, 'I've had a bad day and I lost it.' But you hid it – both of you even given the chance when Ron asked if everything was okay on the job, you denied having problems."

There was a heaviness in the house and in my heart that remains to this day. They went downstairs, packed a few things and piled into their car. I watched from Barry's office window as the car pulled out. Tammy held her head in her hands and leaned against the window. We went to Moose and told her she never had to be frightened again – we had gotten rid of the girls. We asked her if they had hurt her and she said, "Yes." We were so solicitous about her for weeks because of what she had to endure. We couldn't hug and kiss her enough. All of this left me distraught. My support system had collapsed. Who would help us now? Tammy and Rosie had worked for us for one and a half years and lived with us for six months. As far as we were concerned, they were family. We had shared highs and lows; those life cycle events that bind you together until something catastrophic happens to violate that bond.

Chapter XX

GOD SAVED THE BEST FOR LAST

2/98 The task that lay ahead seemed overwhelming. In one month's time, I had to assemble a team of caretakers so I could go with my family to Key West. An SOS went out to everyone who knew our plight and God saved the best for last. We had already hired Maria, the gal from Hospice who bathed Moose three times weekly to come one night a week so we could go out for a few hours. People were so upset when they heard what had happened. The phone began to ring with referrals from nurses and friends of friends who knew people who could help. Over the next week, I set up interviews and called agencies to acquire more help. From now on, there would be no live-in help. We'd have shift work only as needed. I didn't know if I could ever trust myself as a judge of character again. How could I have been so misled? The girls were Christians, quoted scriptures and were successful in totally deceiving us.

Besides Moose, Max was the most victimized. He had grown to love Tammy and Rosie and would go down to their apartment every evening for advice and fellowship. Tammy called to ask forgiveness which was immediate for me. Tammy and Barry are still working on it. We never have heard from Rosie.

One of the volunteers from Hospice said she would

116

do housework for us and quit her job to help out. Another Hospice volunteer told me of his friend who had experience in home care. We hired her, after checking references, to sleep over Saturday evenings so we could get sleep at least one night a week. Moose needed to be checked for dirty or wet diapers and needed to have her position changed to prevent bed sores. Later, I hired a third-year nursing student to sleep over twice a week so we could get uninterrupted sleep.

Another friend of ours, who loved Moose dearly, asked at his church if there were any experienced home-care workers. His pastor recommended one of his flock, Cheryl Walker.

Have you ever instantly liked someone? That's how I felt about Cheryl when she arrived for the interview. I couldn't take my eyes off the wine colored sweater, matching leggings and velvet ballet slippers she wore. We shared the same taste in clothing (hardly criteria for hiring someone, but I hadn't been successful hiring based on qualifications anyhow).

For everyone who keeps on asking receives; and he who keeps on seeking finds; and to him who keeps on knocking, (the door) will be opened. Matthew 6:7

The references I checked gave Cheryl rave reviews. They extolled her ability to take charge, which was exactly what I needed. I was emotionally and physically drained. Cheryl reported to work with a basket of costume jewelry, scarves and other accessories to adorn Moose. After explaining the morning hygiene regime, I left the two alone. Soon I heard music coming from

Moose's room. Cheryl was singing Broadway show tunes. One of her greatest attributes was a lovely voice.

She filled our home with music, humming gospel, pop or whatever moved her that moment.

By her second day on board, Cheryl had indeed taken over the household; and was seeing to Moose's care, as well as overseeing the house cleaning. Soon, the maid paled by comparison to Cheryl, and faded out of the picture.

After one week, I found myself breathing again. By the second week it was as if Cheryl had always been there. The rapid turnover of help until we had stabilized didn't escape Moose. It wasn't easy explaining to her who all these people were who would come and go. Even with all the changes, Moose seemed more relaxed with the girls gone.

Peggy, the nurse, told me of an incident during one of her visits. She was holding Moose's hand after her examination and was about to say good-bye. Moose wouldn't let go of her hand and tried desperately to tell her something, but the words wouldn't come. Peggy, in retrospect, felt Moose had been afraid of the girls and didn't want to be left alone with them.

Chapter XXI

DRESS REHEARSAL

3/98 Several weeks after the girls departed, Moose had another episode. She had been eating so well that I began to feed her regular food cut up into small pieces instead of pureed. One morning, I made her scrambled eggs and sausage. She began to choke and had increased difficulty breathing all day. We suctioned her many times that day. It was similar to that day in December, which prompted us to call in Hospice.

Late that afternoon, the suction machine gave out, and I needed to call the medical supply company to replace the faulty machine. I stepped out of the room to place the call and returned no more than 10 minutes later to find Moose with her head thrown back, her mouth slackened, and her arms hanging limp at her sides. I thought she was dead. I ran through the house calling for Barry, who was in his office. Max and Barry ran with me back to Moose's room. I said, "Do something, please." Barry sprang into action, his physician's skills never too rusty or forgotten. He cleared her passageway and began mouth-to-mouth. I paced. Max ran for his Bible and began reading scriptures out loud holding Moose's hand. I was inept. All I could do was to get on the phone and ask people to pray for Moose. I could not watch.

As I was placing all these calls, a peace came over me. I knew this wasn't going to be it. It couldn't end like this. I called Hospice, who dispatched the nurse on call. I called Chuck, our pastor, who left immediately for our home. In between calls, I'd run back to check on Moose. Max was holding her hand and praying.

We all spoke words of encouragement to her. I remember saying, "Don't be frightened. You're going to be okay." There was no response. Still Barry kept up the mouth-to-mouth. What seemed like light years only amounted to 15 minutes. Finally, as people arrived, the new suction machine was delivered. Barry plugged in the machine and managed to extract a huge glob of mucus that apparently clogged her airway, causing her to expire. She had been cold to the touch and Barry couldn't detect any pulse. She had been dead.

An eternity passed until her eyelids fluttered and she began to breath. Her bedroom was filled with people now. We all stood over her whispering sweet words of encouragement. Soon her labored breathing eased into a more natural rhythm, the color returned to her face. She seemed to be taking it all in. She didn't say anything. The episode took its toll. We didn't know if there would be any brain damage. The nurse arrived and took her vital signs which she said were all strong. It was a miracle and we all rejoiced.

What I said later that evening, after putting her to bed, was that God had put us through a dry run. I was not ready to let go. We all, instinctively, wanted to bring her back and do all that we could to revive her.

For days afterward, I questioned my action – what did I bring her back to? What was the purpose? She was probably already in heaven and we brought her back to pain and suffering – why? But, God had His plan and I was not privy to it. In the meantime, relief washed over me. I was glad to have my mother with me regardless of her impaired condition.

It was a miracle that Barry had been home – I wouldn't have been able to do what he did. In another 10 minutes, he would've left the house to ride his motorcycle on an errand. The passages Max had read were so appropriate for the situation. The suction machine arriving as if on cue, to retrieve the mucus plug, and the prayers offered up on Moose's behalf all contributed to the miracle. She now seemed fine, just tired. All of my strength poured out of me. However, I was thankful to God, for this preview of what was to come. He had been so gracious, allowing me the time I needed to handle the loss. What a loving Father. He knows exactly what I can and can't handle and even provided a dress rehearsal.

I was never more proud of my husband. Perhaps all of his medical training culminated in this triumphant moment – he saved my mother's life that day. I was never more proud of my son. He stood in the face of death and didn't back down. What bravery for a 15-year-old. He was in the trenches and on the front lines with us. I would not want any other people on my team, with the exception of my daughter, who is a great prayer warrior. We had all worked so well together. We were single minded in our purpose that afternoon. Multa corda, una causa (Latin for "many hearts, one cause"). Still, I think nothing can prepare you for that moment when a loved one's soul leaves their body. The finality of it is awesome. I had been so fearful of the death experience.

Psalm 34:4 states; ***I sought the Lord and he delivered me from all my fears.*** From then on, I knew we would all be able to face my mother's death without fear. This was obviously not Moose's time to vacate her earthly body. Not this day, not this time.

Peggy did say, when asked by my brother, that a catastrophic occurrence like this could mark the beginning of the end, which meant two to three months before her body gave out for good. Whatever time Moose had left, I'd count each day and each moment of that day a blessing. We were all stunned.

I prayed it would happen just like that – quickly, without much suffering. How nice if we could design the manner in which we pass from this world into the next.

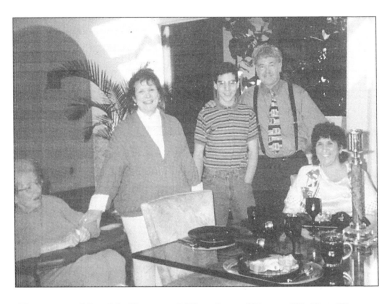

Moose and I, with Max and Chuck and Tresa Miville. These three were a powerful prayer warrior team!

Chapter XXII

A NEEDED BREAK

3/98 Two weeks later with great misgivings, I left for our vacation in Florida. Saying good-bye to Moose was painful for me, since I did not know if I'd see her alive again. Yet, after the trauma of firing the girls and Moose's near death experience, a vacation was not an option anymore, it was a necessity. The team we had assembled was from God. Chuck and Tresa, our pastors, agreed to move into our home and oversee Moose's care. Cheryl moved in as my mother's primary caretaker. Maria came three times a week to bathe Moose and one night for several hours so Cheryl could spend time with her husband and have a break. Pat came one night a week so Cheryl could get some sleep, and a Hospice volunteer came over during the weekends to relieve Cheryl. When I saw how many people it took to fill in for us, it became apparent how much of our time was consumed with Moose's care.

We rented a three bedroom, ocean-front condo in Key West. Brandy and Dirk met us at the airport. Max had his friend Josh join us. It was a deluxe unit with marble floors and a veranda, which faced the ocean running the length of the condo. With the sliding doors open, the sound of waves kissing the shore provided background music. My instructions to everyone were, "Let me sleep. Do not wake me up under penalty of death. I'm not here for sightseeing." I slept until 11:30 a.m. the first day and awakened to muffled conversations from the adjoining living room. It was heavenly. My first thought was to call Moose. She had survived the first day without me. Imagine that! I was reassured that she would be just fine. My main goal was to return home refreshed in body and soul.

Our days were filled with window shopping on the main strip, trying different restaurants, watching the sunsets on the boardwalk with all the street entertainers, vegging out in front of the television, snorkeling and diving for lobsters. Brandy and Dirk caught 16 lobsters on two different dives. What a treat it was to have lobster straight from the ocean to our plates! Max and Josh wanted to try cigar smoking, so I purchased the biggest nastiest cigars for them, in the hopes they would be grossed out. But they loved walking the beaches at night smoking. It made them feel manly. Anyway, the atmosphere was light and breezy and the surroundings were beautiful. I called home each day to talk to Moose, until Cheryl said it wasn't a good idea since Moose would get so upset after speaking to me. I was okay with that as long as I knew she was getting along alright.

The days flew by and soon it was time to say goodbye to Dirk and Brandy. By all accounts, this vacation rated very high on everyone's favorite list. I hated having to leave this heavenly place, but most of all I hated leaving my daughter and son-in-law. We had such a great time hanging out together. We squeezed in as much pleasure out of our time as we could and barely made the airport in time. I knew what we were facing back home – the eventuality of my mother's death. If it weren't for the fact that I missed her so much, I'd be tempted to stay in Florida.

We arrived back home to find Bill, one of the

Hospice volunteers, and Pat, his friend whom he had recommended to come in once a week, sitting side-by-side on the couch. It was only 5:30 p.m. and Moose was put to bed for the evening.

Something about this was not right. Only Pat was supposed to be on duty that day. Moose ordinarily went to bed after dinner at 8 or 9 p.m. After some questioning, it was apparent to me that Moose was put to bed to make life easier on these two. The story was that Pat had injured her foot and Bill was there to help with Moose. After their departure, I went to check on Moose and found that she had soiled herself. I was appalled at the lack of concern the two had shown for Moose.

After some investigation, we fired Pat and reported Bill to Hospice. I know that for the majority of the time Moose had been well cared for. However, on the day of our return (Sunday), Cheryl had gone home after cleaning the house in preparation for our return and had left Moose's care in Pat's hands, as planned. Just those few hours that Moose had been neglected, was too long. It was good to be back. Moose was so happy to see us. We brought her a Key West t-shirt that looked adorable on her. Being back only one day put us right back into the routine. It was as if we had never left. Ten days away was not enough to get caught up on months of interrupted sleep. *(Even after two years, I still have not fully recovered emotionally and physically.)*

Chapter XXIII

THE TRIBUTE

4/98   It was April and spring was upon us. I've always been partial to spring and summer, representing rebirth and watching everything burst into bloom. I'd bring Moose out on the back patio to watch me plant my flower pots and putter in the garden. It was in April that an idea was born. The following month was Max's, Barry's, Cheryl's, and Stan's birthday, as well as Mother's Day. What began as a surprise for everyone's birthday, turned into a celebration honoring Moose for Mother's Day.

I wanted everything to be perfect. There was an overall feeling that this was to be my last Mother's Day with her. She was dying. How could I make this special? Alzheimer's had stolen my 83-year-old mother's life, piece by piece, leaving a fragile, wheelchair-bound woman, who spent the majority of her days muttering unintelligible sounds. Even if she couldn't grasp what was going on, I decided that a living tribute to celebrate her life seemed most appropriate. I would have one final opportunity to honor the person she had been. Most memorials, I realized, occur after death. But, I wanted to recount her virtues while she could still hear what I had to say.

It seemed important to let people involved in her life to realize that she once was a vital, intelligent, prolific writer and communicator before the onset of this debilitating disease. That was the mother I remembered.

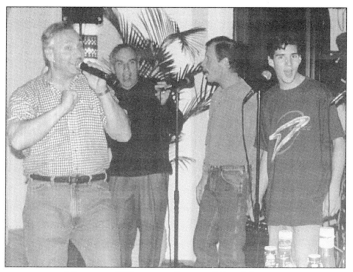

Now and Then performed for Moose.

The house that night was alive with laughter. Clusters of people dotted the interior. Staff members from Hospice of the Comforter chatted with Moose's other caregivers, along with nurses and devoted friends. In her most incapacitated state, Moose had managed to capture the hearts of many people.

That night, Moose was at the center of it all. She looked radiant – almost regal. We'd selected a black beaded gown for her to wear. Her naturally curly, white hair provided a magnificent frame for a flawless complexion. Even her nails were freshly polished. Although it didn't matter to her, we fussed over her like a prom queen.

The weather may have been stormy outside, but the warm, festive atmosphere inside, compensated. Music filled the air with '50s tunes sung by *Now And Then*. Because Moose had been their most loyal fan, attending every rehearsal and performance, they gladly consented to entertain us. With every detail of the

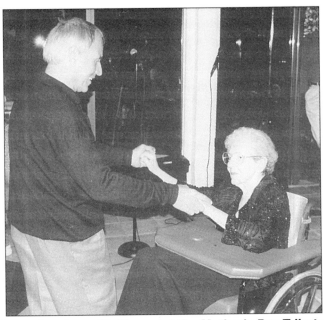

Barry dancing with Moose at the Mother's Day Tribute.

evening carefully planned, I was ready to watch it unfold.

I had cooked for days. The table was laden with delectable goodies and adorned with flowers, flanked by candles. Glancing around the room, I realized it was time to begin. So, I approached the microphone and began reminiscing. I talked of her childhood, her marriage, her triumphs and sorrows. Moose sat in rapt attention as I recounted her struggles through the years. I ended by thanking her for the privilege of escorting her to the end of her road, and presented her with a dozen yellow roses.

Had any of this penetrated her dark world? No one knows for sure. She hadn't called me by name in over a year, but just then, she reached her hand toward me and whispered softly, "Fran, Fran." She would be gone in just one short month, but I have that memory forever. It was her Mother's Day gift to me.

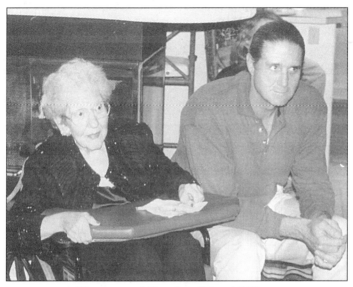

Moose and "her boyfriend," Stan.

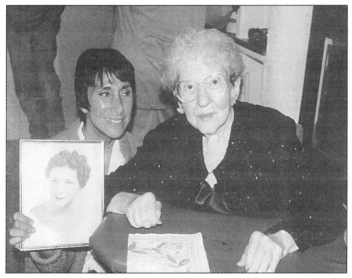

Maria, with Moose, at the Mother's Day Tribute.

Chapter XXIV

THE FINAL CURTAIN

6/98 It was a Sunday like any other. Dragging myself out of bed, I staggered into Moose's room at dawn. I'd always round the corner and peek into her room to see if her shoulders were moving, indicating she was still alive. Gwen reported that Moose had a restless night. She had already given her the morning meds and prepared her for church. I told Gwen that she could leave after she dressed Moose and put her back in bed until the Hospice volunteer arrived to feed her breakfast.

I left to get myself ready for home church. When Janice arrived, I informed her of Moose's restless night,

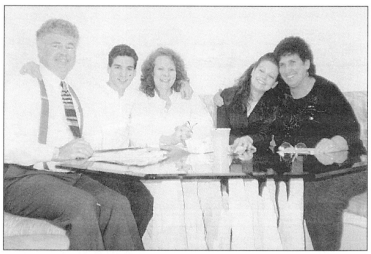

Our pastors, Chuck and Tresa Miville (on left and right), started coming to the house Sunday mornings so we could have church with Moose. Max, myself, and the Miville's daughter, are seated in center.

and told her to watch for any signs of congestion. Moose's breakfast, these days, consisted of a power drink, cream of wheat or scrambled eggs. The routine was to bring Moose's breakfast to her bedroom. Janice would feed her while I finished dressing. Then I'd return to see how Moose was doing.

Janice expressed concern – Moose wasn't eating well and was gurgling – a sign of congestion. I asked if she could deep suction Moose. I had an attachment to the normal suction machine capable of reaching deep into the lungs and removing phlegm. Since Janice was a nurse, I felt comfortable with her ability to perform this procedure. Something told me we needed it today. Janice cautioned me that Moose would be tired out from this procedure and it could stimulate more production of fluids in the lungs. I needed to take the chance, as we'd have no help scheduled for the rest of the day and taking an aggressive stand seemed to be the right thing to do. Janice, sensing Moose's condition could become serious, gave me her home phone number in the event she needed more suctioning.

The Mivilles arrived for church and we brought Moose in for the service. Moose seemed agitated and worn out at the same time. Once services began, my mother gratefully drifted off to sleep. I kept watching her. Something was wrong. I didn't like how she was slouched in her wheelchair. After services, I invited Chuck and Tresa to cool off in the pool. We rolled Moose outside to get some fresh air and sunshine. All the while, I kept a watchful eye on her breathing. She didn't look well. Her face was ashen. I commented to Tresa that I was concerned. We could be going into another episode like the day Moose had died, months earlier. Would I be ready to let her go?

After the Mivilles left, we offered to take Moose for a ride – she loved that so much. It always seemed to elevate her spirits. She wasn't too talkative that day, rather withdrawn, actually. We loaded her in the car and took Max for his guitar lesson. It began to pour. There was thunder and lightening. We drove around because it seemed to keep Moose calmed down. Before picking Max up from his lesson, we stopped to get a pizza for dinner. Moose had fallen asleep. I was grateful for the naps as I knew she was getting the rest that her frail body needed for restoration.

Moose just had a light dinner that night because the nurse said her throat would be sore from the procedure. Again, she was restless. I got up frequently that night to check on her.

I was always thankful for Monday – it meant reinforcements would arrive to help with Moose. It would be Cheryl's last day before leaving for three days. I gave her a report on Moose's bad day. She got Moose up and dressed as usual. Moose had revived. I fixed her the powdered protein concoction with tofu, frozen berries and a banana. She had to have been hungry because she didn't eat much on Sunday. Cheryl reported, "Moose said, 'This is shit'," referring to the drink. These understandable outbursts were always a surprise, as most of what she said was inaudible.

I replied, "Just make sure she gets liquids in her. We don't want her to get dehydrated. We'll try giving her juice later." We needed to get calories in her. I was always afraid of her losing weight. Cheryl turned on the TV for her. Her color had returned and she was looking better. I didn't tell Cheryl I was apprehensive about her leaving for a few days, even though Emily, her replacement, was quite competent.

Later, for lunch, she ate crackers, tuna and jello. I was elated. She was back on track, her appetite having returned. We still had to decide if we should keep our social engagement that night. Parents of one of Max's classmates, Ashley, had invited us all to dinner. I wasn't sure if it was wise to take Moose out, but as the day progressed I felt more confident about her condition. Whenever there was an upcoming event, I'd tell Moose about it so she would have something to look forward to. I observed Moose all day to look for any sign that the congestion had returned. I would've cancelled dinner or sent Max and Barry, while I stayed home with Moose. But she seemed like she was back to her old self and looking forward to going out. I felt secure in the fact that we lived just minutes from Ashley and could take Moose home if she was not feeling well.

We arrived for dinner and Ashley's family made us feel very comfortable and they were especially welcoming to Moose, that my fears were allayed. It was a lovely evening and Moose seemed to be enjoying all the attention they lavished on her. She sat with us at the table and like a hungry animal, kept reaching for food. I was afraid to give her too much because of how ill she had been the previous day. Not knowing how Moose was going to respond in a social situation made me edgy. But that night, other than reaching for food, she was fine. After feeding her, I asked if she could watch TV in another room. It gave me a chance to relax and participate in the conversation without constantly watching Moose. We had a lively discussion about multi-level marketing and a good time in general. Every so often, I'd check on

Moose. Part of me felt guilty, letting her sit by herself. I never really knew what Moose was thinking or feeling. There was no barometer. I would just whisper to her that it wouldn't be too much longer before we'd leave for home. In retrospect, if I hurt Moose's feelings in any way, I'd be distraught. But comparing her life to the activity level of people shuffled off to nursing homes, whose relatives visit them on an average of 15 minutes a week, I felt assured that she had the highest quality of life possible for someone in the advanced stages of this disease.

The next day (Tuesday) would be Emily's first day on the job. Emily was punctual and eager to jump in. I helped her get Moose up and dressed to show her the morning regimen. Emily had cared for her aging aunt until she died and through that experience had gained knowledge and compassion to care for others.

Moose was not 100%. I supposed she would be very hungry by now. I made her a power shake and cream of wheat. She had a little of each. That day we would be visited by Rita, the social worker from Hospice. She was to assess Moose's ability to travel as Reuben had requested. It seemed absurd for Moose, in her condition, to go visit him at his newly acquired home in Wisconsin.

By the time Rita arrived, Moose was slouched in her wheelchair, a posture she assumed if she wasn't doing well. I kept pulling her up to a sitting position, to no avail. Concerned, I called Peggy, the nurse, to make sure she would stop by and check on Moose. Upon seeing her, Rita determined on the spot that if Reuben wanted to see Moose, he'd have to travel to Colorado, not the reverse. Rita said she would inform Reuben of Moose's condition and recommend he come out for a visit.

By the time Peggy arrived, Moose was congested. I suggested to Peggy, she do the deep suctioning like we did on Sunday. I told her Moose had had a bad day Sunday, but rallied on Monday. Peggy obliged me, cautioning that suctioning only provided temporary relief. I agreed but said that I couldn't stand to hear her gurgling and choking. After performing the procedure, she commented that Moose had not offered any resistance to the tube going down her throat, meaning that she had lost the gag reflex. The ramifications of this being, that anything fed to her could go into the lungs causing pneumonia. Her vital signs, usually strong, were not good. Her blood pressure was low and her heart beat fast, meaning the heart was working hard to circulate the blood. Peggy gently informed me that the dying process had begun. I asked if this process had ever been reversed. She told me a story about one of her former patients. Hospice had contacted his daughter, whom he hadn't seen in years. She decided to come visit her dying father. Once he heard his daughter was coming, he arose from the deathbed, dressed and wanted to be clean shaven. They had a wonderful visit. He died shortly after she left.

Part of me refused to believe this could be it for Moose. She had rallied so many times before. Peggy asked if she should inform Reuben of Moose's condition. I said, "Of course." Before leaving, she cautioned me to be very careful what I fed Moose. Max was working at Billy's Pizza. I called and asked him to bring home some of Billy's homemade ices and chicken soup.

That day and the following two days, Moose's boyfriend, Stan, came to visit her. Moose met Stan when we took her to church to hear a preacher talk on healing. At the end, we took Moose up to the altar for prayer. When we looked up, there was a wall of a man praying fervently for Moose. Stan was 6'6", dressed in biking leathers with a pony tail trailing down his back. He was the president of Bikers for Jesus. From that day on, there was a spiritual alliance between Moose and Stan. He would visit Moose regularly and pray for her. He gave her a picture that she would hold all day. Once she was able to blurt out, "He's a big, big man and I love him." Cheryl had informed him that Moose had a bad day on Sunday. When he arrived, it was apparent that Moose wasn't doing well. He pulled me aside to say she didn't look good. My head was agreeing but my heart was believing she'd pull through as always.

When Max returned with the food, I fed Moose with a sponge-tipped applicator. She was dehydrated and welcomed the cool refreshing ices. There was fear in her eyes. I tried to be upbeat and reassuring for her sake as well as my own. Fortunately, it was Tuesday and Gwen was coming that night so we could get some sleep. I felt beaten up. This roller coaster ride was taking its emotional toll on us. I was happy to pass the baton to Gwen. Before turning in for the night, I recognized that Moose was feverish. Peggy prescribed Tylenol® in suppository form, so we knew it would get into Moose's system.

In the following days, Moose would hang onto people's hands for dear life – a death-grip. I think she felt if she let go that she'd just slip away. I put cold compresses on her head and spoke softly to her.

Wednesday was another bad day. We kept Moose in clean bed clothes and as comfortable as possible. We didn't put her dentures in. I didn't want to add to her distress. The days were a blur. I didn't even remember getting dressed or functioning. I felt like I had cried an ocean of tears, yet I hadn't shed one. My sockets hurt. I was desperate not to have this a reality, but if this was going to be the finale, let it be over soon. I couldn't take a prolonged good-bye. My prayer for my mother was that she would go peacefully in her sleep, not drowning in phlegm. Stan came again as did other friends. It was a relief to talk to people. We tried to carry on as usual. Barry even counselled three people while Max continued going to work. He was travailing over Moose and could not sleep well. He'd come into our room to be with us. One night neither of us could sleep. We went into the living room and talked. I told him this was probably the end and the toughest part of our journey with Moose. He was visibly upset, but like me, he didn't show his emotions or talk about it too much.

Wednesday night, Barry and I were on duty. We decided to sleep in Moose's hospital bed to keep close watch over her. We thought it best to have her in the recliner, propped up, to assist her breathing. Barry kept suctioning her. At 2:00 a.m. I couldn't take listening to her labored breathing anymore. I went into our bedroom. Gratefully, I fell asleep. At 6:30 a.m. Barry came in to tell me that Moose was resting comfortably and that he successfully suctioned up a lot of phlegm. I went to see for myself. She did indeed look much better. There was something comforting about checking on her and seeing her little face with sunken cheeks and no teeth. She was alive.

Emily came prepared to make some chicken soup. After all, chicken soup had saved her once before. Emily was encouraging. We decided to believe it possible for Moose to come back from the edge – as she had so many times before. Emily kept bringing supplies from home that her aunt had used: a special air mattress to prevent bed sores, a vaporizer with medicine for the lungs and a potent ointment for sore spots. She was a veritable storehouse of information and cache of medical reserves. I will always refer to her as a low flying angel, one of many, God sent to minister to Moose.

Thursday morning Peggy was off duty, but she requested the on-call nurse check on Moose. Emily and I got Moose up, sponge-bathed her, and put clean clothes on her. We anxiously awaited the nurse's report after examining Moose. Once again, God granted us a miracle! Her blood pressure had returned to normal, her heart slowed down and her lungs sounded fairly clear, with the exception of some crackling in one lobe. Emily and I were elated. We believed the worst was over and once again, my mother had cheated death. We were ready to begin the slow steady road back to health. We'd try feeding Moose.

Rita called later that day to say Reuben declined the invitation to visit Moose, but said that he would like to speak to her. So we arranged for Rita to come at 4:00 p.m. the next day, when we would place a call to Reuben and hold the receiver to Moose's ear.

Stan came around noon and was overjoyed to see Moose up and with it. He said he was wrong about Moose's condition and felt she would make it. We were all in a celebrative mood. I asked Moose if she would like to go for a ride. She replied, as usual, "Let's go." I pureed the chicken soup and fed it to her on the sponge appli-cator with some of Billy's ices.

After lunch, Barry, Max and I happily piled into the car with Moose. I remember looking at Barry and both of us saying what a relief it was to have Moose doing better. We went shopping in a department store. Moose seemed content just to be hanging out with us. The feeling was mutual. It was a beautiful day and we were exhausted but relieved that the crisis had passed. We came home and pushed Moose's wheelchair out by the pool to get some sunshine and fresh air on her. After Barry and I had eaten, I fed Moose some applesauce and ices to hydrate her. The food was oozing out the side of her mouth. I attributed it to her either forgetting how to swallow, or her throat being too sore from all the suctioning. In any case, I decided to try feeding her again later. Tonight, Maria was scheduled to come from 7 to 10 p.m. Barry and I, in lieu of going out, would catch up on our sleep while Maria watched Moose.

One thing Moose and I enjoyed doing after dinner, was to return to her bedroom to watch *Entertainment Tonight* together. I had bought my mother a card for Mother's Day but misplaced it. That day I spied it in a box of Vedalia onions. I was happy to get the chance to read it to Moose. It had such meaning to be able to tell her how much she meant to us having just faced the threat of losing her. I read the card to her, showering her with hugs and kisses. We looked at family pictures and talked about each person. It was a special time.

When Maria arrived, I gave her the change-of-shift report and asked her to try and get some food down Moose. She was delighted to see her doing better. I told her we'd be in the next room resting, if she needed anything. It would be the last time Moose and I could talk to each other.

I checked on Moose several times that night. She seemed to be resting comfortably. Barry got up Friday morning to feed the pets. He came back in to report that Moose was still sleeping. I wanted to see for myself. As I rounded the corner of Moose's room, I paused a moment to focus on her shoulders to see if she was breathing, she was. Relieved, I came around the bed to see her cute little face. She was always happy to see me in the morning, or maybe she was just happy to be alive. I would try to greet her in an upbeat way like, "Good morning, sleepy head. Are you ready to get up?" Something inside told me to let her sleep that day. Cheryl would be returning today. Although Emily was terrific, there was something comforting about getting back to normal, as if this would help Moose get back her health.

Peggy, concerned about Moose, came to take her vital signs. She basically said that things had not been reversed and Moose's body was still shutting down. She prescribed morphine in case she exhibited signs of distress. She instructed me to let Moose stay in bed as her body was tired. I knew she was right.

Barry, on the other hand, even with all his medical training, was in denial, saying Moose had entered a new phase – staying in bed all the time. But I knew this was the end. I didn't know how long it would take, but God had prepared my heart for this time. I was ready.

I decided it was time to call relatives and let them know the situation was grave. I phoned Lucille, Moose's 80-year-old sister in Texas, who was still grieving over her husband's death, a year prior to this. She seemed to be in denial as well. I could only inform – it wasn't my job to handle everyone's grief for them. It was all I could do to keep myself strong and clear-headed. The next call was to Brandy, my daughter. She and Dirk were going on a qualifying dive for their Divemaster certification. I reported that Moose's health was declining and they should try to keep in touch over the weekend. She felt helpless, wanting to be with us, but having been launched into her own life, she had responsibilities there. Lastly, I phoned Moose's cousins, Mort and Judy, in California. They were about to leave on a trip. I told them I would keep them posted and leave messages for them.

Having taken care of that, I could get back to Moose. Cheryl had called the night before. I didn't want her to be shocked at seeing Moose after her three day hiatus. When she arrived, we walked into Moose's room. Things were quiet. We all fell into taking care of our chores, moving silently around the house. Peggy returned to check on Moose, bringing Barbra Streisand's new CD. She thought there were some songs I could get strength from. We set up a mobile CD player in Moose's room and played the CD for her. We kept cool cloths on Moose's head and I spoke softly to her. I opened the curtains so she could see the beautiful blooming flowers I'd planted on her balcony. I asked Cheryl to stay longer so Barry and I could get some rest. Cheryl sat beside Moose and sang hymns to her. People came and went all day.

I was preoccupied. We decided to get Moose up at 3:00. I wanted her to be alert for Reuben's call. We freshened her up and sat her in the recliner. I told her Reuben wanted to talk to her. She was non-communicative saying "lalalalalala" in low tones. Rita and Peggy came at the appointed time. Barry and I had discussed listening in on Reuben's call, to abort anything inappropriate he might say to her by hanging up. I didn't want to give him a last chance to disrespect her. We decided not to eavesdrop as whatever he said to her would be between them and God.

We assembled in Moose's room and placed the call. Rita asked if she was ready and placed the phone up to Moose's ear. There was no observable response or change in my mother's demeanor while Reuben spoke, saying only "lalalala." Rita, after a few minutes, took the receiver and asked if Reuben was finished, to which he replied "yes." Peggy then walked out of the room with the phone to report to him about Moose's condition. Their conversation was brief. Peggy said he wanted to know why we weren't feeding her through IVs or a tube inserted in the stomach. Peggy said this had been Moose's wish not to be kept alive via artificial means or heroic measures. Meanwhile, I told Moose that Reuben had called and that he loved her and wanted to speak to her.

There was no response. We put her back in bed. Everyone left and a quiet fell over the household.

I called Chuck and Tresa, our pastors, and told them of Moose's condition. They came right over. I don't remember how I passed the time. I only felt an extreme heaviness in my spirit. My body kept going like a well-oiled machine but I wore fatigue and sorrow like overcoats. I couldn't shake it. The first thing Tresa said when she arrived was that God told her to wash my hair. Even though it was clean, I acquiesced. She said she just wanted to do this for me. Truth be known, it felt wonderful and soothing to have someone fussing with my hair. Barry and Chuck sat outside by the pond talking quietly. To this day, I don't know what they talked about.

After washing my hair, Tresa and I sat by the fireplace in the kitchen as night began to fall. After their arrival, an unexplainable peace descended over our home – an extraordinary peace that still exists. It is this peace that sustained me and continues to do so through everything. I felt like God was wanting me to rest in Him. As Tresa and I spoke, a lovely scent of flowers permeated the air. Only I could smell it. I said, "Hey, isn't a sign of the Lord's presence – a sweet scent?" She said, "Yes, I feel the presence of the Lord, He is here."

We decided to go into Moose's room. It was twilight and a soft breeze was coming through the door to her balcony. Moose was resting peacefully. I had Tresa sit in the recliner chair next to the bed while I played Barbra Streisand's CD. I laid on the floor and we quietly listened to the music. Tresa said that Moose was on her own journey now – in God's hands. It was out of my control. My job was over. We listened without another word spoken. The breeze, peace and music made that evening magical.

When we got to the song, *Standing On Holy Ground*, and particularly the phrase, "There are angels all around," I stood up and danced. I could feel angels in that room that night. Moose was indeed on her way to meeting the Lord. There was a transition taking place. God had lifted the burden from my shoulders. I was released. I was free. There was nothing left for me to do as caregiver, except keep Moose company as she departed. I could do that. I would see this journey through from beginning to end. I felt God was answering another prayer by allowing Moose to gently slip away peacefully.

If you live in Me and My words remain in you and continue to live in your hearts, ask whatever you will, and it shall be done for you. John 15:7

Barry and Chuck joined us in listening to the music. It was dark now. Peace reigned from that night on. It was my most spiritual moment ever. What a privilege for us to be with my mother now, watching as she gave herself over to death. There was no travailing, no pain, no need for drugs. Everything that had taken place before was preparing me to relinquish her now.

Peace I leave with you; My peace I now give and bequeath to you. Not as the world gives do I give to you. Do not let your hearts be troubled, neither let them be afraid. John 14:27

Chuck and Tresa left us in a more tranquil state than when they had arrived. I was grateful. I'm always grateful when someone does something for us. I was so accustomed to helping others. God had been good to us, placing us in a position to lend our expertise to others whether it was counselling or financial aid. Now I was in need and it was okay to receive help from others around us. I allowed myself this – why not? If someone could ease my pain, relieve my burden, why not let them?

Although we were at peace, we were physically and emotionally exhausted and slept soundly that night. Barry, as usual, got up early. He reported that Moose was sleeping soundly. I checked for myself. It seemed that her heart was working hard. All I could do was keep her clean and comfortable. I opened her curtains so she could see out. Her eyes were opened but not focused. As I spoke, her eyes tried to follow the sound. They were glazed over and mechanical like photo lenses. At one point, she was staring up at the corner of her room. I said, "Moose what do you see? Are there angels here for you?" She didn't answer. I believe she was on the threshold between this life and the next. I busied myself, straightening things around her room until Cheryl arrived. She was my rock. I left the room to get dressed and cleaned up after Cheryl came.

We were like a tag team. Moose was never left alone that day. I made arrangements to go out with some friends to get away from the "death watch." I didn't know how I'd be feeling, actually. Gwen would sleep over so we could get some rest. None of us knew this would be Moose's last day with us.

The countdown had begun without our permission. At one point, I went into Moose's room, held her in my arms and told her I was going to miss her, and to please give me a sign when she crossed over to the other side, that she was okay. I stroked her head and sat by her bed in the reclining chair watching television. I read Psalm 23 to her.

We listened to the Streisand CD as I made a list of people to inform of Moose's death. People came and went. Hours passed without me noticing. Max and Barry were going to be on the radio that night. Barry came in and suggested that I should leave the room, but I didn't want to. So instead, he came in to keep me company. I wanted to do something to honor him. I sat on the floor and washed his feet. It was late afternoon.

Moose's life was slipping away and I didn't know what to do with mine. She didn't seem to be in any discomfort, thank God. I kept her mouth moist, her brow cool and her bottom dry. My responsibility was coming to an end. I couldn't even allow myself to think what I'd do with my life after she was gone.

At 5:30 p.m., Max and Barry left for the radio

station for their monthly Christian radio talk show for teens. Soon after our friends came over. We decided to order food in instead of eating out. Food was the last thing on my mind. I just wanted the fellowship. It was comforting having other people around. They were able to momentarily distract me from the "death watch." By 7:00 p.m., Gwen had arrived to start the evening shift, allowing me to relax a little. Shortly afterward, Barry and Max returned. We ordered food in and managed to have a few laughs, although I wanted to jump up and check on Moose every 10 to 15 minutes. Barry was cracking jokes. Meanwhile, a foreboding thunderstorm provided the background mood for the evening. Our attempts to keep everything light and breezy, were just that. I remember thinking to myself, the chariots were coming for Moose. As the evening wore on, fatigue overtook me and I was relieved when our friends left at 10:00 p.m. My eyelids felt like they were 1,000 pounds apiece. Before turning in, I stopped for the last time to check on Moose. Gwen said nothing had changed.

I kissed Moose on the forehead and held her hand, not knowing what morning would bring. I instructed Gwen to please wake us up if there was any change. My head hit the pillow and I lapsed into a deep sleep, although I could hear Max rattling around in the kitchen. I wanted to get up and tell him to get some rest but I was paralyzed from exhaustion.

I awakened to Gwen, softly calling my name. Instinctively, I jumped up. A thousand things raced through my head. She reported that she had given my mother a breathing treatment, which seemed to give Moose temporary relief, but then she had gasped for air and stopped breathing. We all ran for her bedroom. I looked at Moose lying on her back, her mouth slightly ajar, her eyes vacant and her chest and shoulders still. I felt her chest with my hand; there was no movement.

I said, "I do believe that she is gone." Barry asked if I wanted him to do anything.

I replied, "No, it's over, she's at peace now, leave her be." A strange calm took over me. I was on automatic pilot. Barry wept for a few minutes while I kicked into gear. Gwen seemed to be in shock. She had not ever lost a patient before. I thanked her and said there was nothing more she could've done. "Don't blame yourself," I whispered in her ear. She turned off the oxygen and I had her help me put Moose into a warm, long night-gown.

I asked to be alone with my mother. I took her flaccid arm and put it around me as I bent down for the last time to kiss her. It was a throwback to childhood. Even in death I had to ask for affection. I told her I would miss seeing her elf-like face everyday and that she had done the best job she knew how as a mother. I hugged her and left the room.

I escorted Gwen to the door with my arm around her. It was 2:30 a.m. We called, as instructed, Hospice of the Comforter. The procedure was to have the nurse on call come and declare the patient dead. Max, Barry and I sat in the kitchen talking, awaiting the nurse's arrival.

It was that eerie time of day, not quite morning yet. The storm had abated and it was quiet in the house. We talked to Max. I asked him why he was up. He said that he couldn't sleep. He had been travailing over Moose. The nurse arrived, offered condolences, then proceeded to Moose's room. She listened with a stethoscope for a heartbeat.

They have to listen for a prescribed period of time before officially declaring a person dead. For a second, I thought what a fluke it would be if she once again cheated death and began to breathe. That was not the case. The nurse, taking the stethoscope from her ears said, "She is gone." We went back into the kitchen where she asked which mortuary was to be called. She placed a call to them.

She then asked If I wanted my brother to be called now. I said yes. I listened as she said "Reuben, this is Carol, from Hospice of the Comforter. I'm calling to tell you that Maxine, your mother, has just passed away." She paused, apparently waiting for a response, and then replied, "A half hour ago." Then she asked him, "Do you have any other questions for me at this time?" They said their good-byes and she hung up the receiver.

We sat in the kitchen chatting until the people from the mortuary arrived. There were some papers to sign and I excused myself returning to my bedroom. I couldn't bear to see them removing my mother in a body bag. As I went into our darkened bedroom, God spoke, "Job well-done." Then a strange thing occurred. My right hand began to itch terribly. Slowly, I realized this must be a sign from Moose. Her palms used to itch occasionally. I knew it was her saying, "It's okay. I'm fine." I smiled and got into bed and waited for Barry to join me. Oddly enough, we were all able to go back to sleep until dawn.

We called Chuck and Tresa who said they'd be over shortly. We decided not to have a traditional funeral service but to plan Moose's memorial service ourselves. I placed calls to my aunt, my daughter, my cousins and Barry's parents. It was Father's Day, June 21st, and I didn't want to stay home. I knew we needed to get out. We called our friends, the DeSalvos, a large Italian family we'd known for years. They said, "Come over, the whole family is going to be here." That was perfect. They lived 40 minutes away and it was a beautiful drive through the country. After the perfunctory calls were made, I jumped into the shower and got dressed. It was an odd feeling to be parentless – an unexplainable feeling. When Chuck and Tresa arrived, we started planning the memorial service.

Afterward, we headed for the DeSalvo's and a Father's Day celebration. It was the right thing to do. There was an air of festivity. The DeSalvos have five children and eight grandchildren of all ages. Kids were everywhere. One by one, family members came up and hugged me offering condolences. I held babies and schmoozed with everyone. It was as if life was starting again for me. Max needed diversion too. Tony, the DeSalvo's youngest, grew up with Max. Something told me that celebrating Father's Day this way began our healing. As festive as that day was, when the three of us returned to our large, empty house, it felt like a tomb.

The following day, I would kick into high gear planning and executing my mother's memorial service.

In the weeks and months ahead, I would never once think I'd heard my mother's voice, or jump out of bed to check on her, or catch myself going down the aisles in the grocery store looking for her specialty foods. I believe God gave me instant healing from everything. How good He is!

Chapter XXV

THE MEMORIAL SERVICE

The week between Moose's death and her memorial service was spent in a frantic effort to plan a meaningful farewell for my mother. I was grateful to be able to focus on the event not the loss. I wanted the service to reflect a perfect blend of her relaxed style and natural class. She was not a pretentious woman, nor was she religious, although she spoke often of a God who was always watching out for her. That became the underlying theme. A month prior to her death, God gave me a vision to have the service at home where she lived and died.

A transformation began taking place in the household. I instructed Cheryl to dismantle Moose's room – to return the rented equipment to clear out the evidence of an ailing person. Moose was in another place now, whole again.

I had not gone back into her room since her body had been removed. There was a funny feeling in the pit of my stomach whenever I was near her room. Finally, Cheryl took me by the hand and said, "Are you ready?" Not knowing for sure if I was but wanting to get it over, I answered, "Sure let's do it." When we went into the room, I knew that everything would be okay. Things were slowly disappearing; the porta-potty, the bed and mattress, the oxygen tanks, the suction machine and all her medications from the bathroom counter. I could still feel the peace that descended over the house the Friday

Moose slipped into a comatose state. I knew then that this room would be my haven where I would write about our journey.

The linens had been taken to the laundry to be washed. I asked Cheryl to retrieve the pillow cases and put them back on my mother's pillows. I put them to my face and could smell her. Some might think this morbid, but I found it comforting to be able to capture her essence in a pillow. I told Cheryl to have the wheelchair picked up after the memorial service. I had something in mind for it.

Her clothes would be stored in her closet for later disposition. While Cheryl attended to those details, I addressed writing the obituary, selecting the picture for it, and making sure it would appear in the Chicago papers so life-long friends would be notified.

I contacted Carol, who arranged for the sisterhood at Temple to cater the food. After speaking to the mortuary about printing programs, I dropped off a suggested format. Although we would allot time for anyone who wanted to speak, I approached several people to participate in the memorial, such as our pastor, who would talk about the significance of the Father, calling Moose home on Father's Day, and Stan, the man who lit up Moose's life for the last nine months, and Dick Polinsky, the former president of the Temple Shalom, to lead us in Kaddish, the Jewish mourner's prayer. Cheryl agreed to sing *My Life Is In Your Hands*, the song she had rehearsed for my mother's tribute, but due to illness was unable to perform. How perfect for her to do it now. And, all the while, I was rehearsing the eulogy.

I personally placed calls to invite people, arrange for a harpist, order garden chairs, order delicatessen trays from Denver, order flowers, and to arrange the music. John, a member of Barry and Max's singing group, and another of Moose's boyfriends agreed to help with the music. I selected two songs from Streisand's CD: *Standing On Holy Ground* and *Avinu Malkeinu,* a Hebrew song, asking God to forgive our sins and to show mercy.

Each day I would dash about with a list of things to accomplish: blow up a picture of Moose to poster size to be mounted, print copies of the Hebrew prayer to be inserted in the programs, find words to the songs, stop at the Temple Shalom to get the words to Hebrew prayers, pick up candy and sodas. The list seemed endless.

But everything was falling into place. Fruit baskets began to appear. Cards, phone calls, flower arrangements, and homemade goodies were left at our doorstep. Inspirational tapes, books, dinners and donations in my mother's memory, flooded our home. We were enveloped in love and peace.

Brandy, who wanted to be with us desperately, struggled with whether or not she should come. There were calls back and forth. We told her that if she was coming for our benefit, she should stay home. But, if she needed closure for herself, then she should come. She had to determine this for herself. She finally decided to stay home, since we would be coming to see her three days after the service. I gave her a detailed account of the plans and even had Cheryl sing over the phone to her. I also asked Josh, Max's friend, to video the service and direct traffic. The days were filled with exacting details, and by Thursday, all the arrangements were completed.

Barry suggested that we take advantage of a gift certificate that Brandy and Dirk had given us to a lovely fondue restaurant for our anniversary. At first, I thought we should wait for a better time, but then I realized this was a special time. I needed to slow down and spend some time with just my husband, who had been a tremendous support to my mother and was mourning her loss as well.

We put the top down on my car and took a leisurely drive to the restaurant. It was a welcome relief from a hectic week to luxuriate for hours over a sumptuous meal. I realized for the first time, that we needn't rush home to relieve a nurse. From now on we had all the time in the world. We also noted how long it had been since we visited this part of town, as we strolled back to the car after dinner. This would be the first observations of change since Moose's departure. There would be others.

At last, Sunday arrived. My biggest concern was weather – this is always a consideration when an event is planned outdoors. Cheryl bounced in to do a last minute clean-up job. She informed me the weather girl announced there was absolutely no chance for rain – an answer to prayer. Carol and the sisterhood team arrived on time and promptly took over the kitchen. White chairs were delivered and set up in the garden. The florist arrived with the magnificent cream and white colored floral table arrangement and a huge similar spray to be displayed on a stand next to my mother's picture, in the entry.

I had a special gardenia wreath designed that I placed in front of a picture of Moose, Brandy and I on the seat of her vacant wheelchair. This would be parked on the veranda where speeches would be made. John came early to set up the speakers, microphone and sound system. I took some quiet time to compose my thoughts. Meanwhile, the harpist arrived and set up on the upper terrace. She was hired to play while guests arrived until the service began. Stan called that morning to ask if it was okay to dress in his motorcycle leathers. I told him that Moose would love it. I wanted everyone to do and say what was on their hearts. I provided the framework and atmosphere, God would do the rest.

Cheryl had gifted me with a long black dress with sequins around the neck because it matched a black blazer I owned. I knew the minute she gave it to me, I would save it for my mother's memorial. I had spoken earlier to Brandy and told her the content of my eulogy. She cautioned me to take my time and say everything on my heart – don't rush it. I wanted this to be a perfect day for Moose.

Outside, the harp music played softly. It was heavenly. The garden was a profusion of color, attracting beautiful butterflies. There was a soft breeze blowing providing relief from the sun's glorious rays, and the sound of water splashing into the pond was soothing. This natural outdoor setting was more apropos than a stuffy chapel where Moose had never been. It was she who watched over my shoulder as I planted all these flowers and watered them daily. Now they were giving back to her.

Cheryl, who had struggled all week with a sore throat, approached the microphone and began "My Life Is In Your Hands." A hush spread throughout the audience. I've never heard her sing more beautifully than that moment. She was anointed. The wind carried her voice and it was powerful. Barry began to sob.

There was silence when she finished. The moment I had rehearsed was at hand. I kicked off my shoes and began my mother's eulogy by saying, "There wa no question that Moose's life was in the Lord's hands," and that "He orchestrated a symphony of people to accompany her through the valley of the shadow of death." This time, now, was meant to acknowledge those people who spent time with Moose from the onset of Alzheimer's to the end. It was a chronicle of her last years punctuated with poignant poems, pictures and anecdotes, marking her descent into silence. I ended with the following Jewish prayer, which I personalized for her:

When I Think Of You

Whenever there is a spectacular sunrise or sunset, leaving the sky ablaze, I will think of you.

When I see buds on all the trees and explosions of colored blooms marking the passage of spring, I will think of you.

When I hear the laughter of children frolicking on a summer's day, I will think of you.

When the leaves turn colors and rustle by an open window and there's a crispness to the air, I will think of you.

When the snow silently blankets the earth and glistens in the moonlight, I will think of you.

In the beginning of the year and when it ends, I will think of you.

When I am weary and in need of strength, I will think of you.

When I am lost and sick at heart, I will think of you.

When there are celebrations I yearn to share, I will think of you.

So long as I live, you too shall live for you are now a part of me as I think of you.

Moose had taught me a final and most important lesson in life, how to love and be loved without saying a word.

Following my eulogy, Stan Plesinski got up and gave an impassioned plea to those who were unsaved to dedicate their lives to the Lord, as he believed Moose had done. He said that he knew he would see Moose again, as we who believe all will.

Dick Polinsky then led the congregation in the mourner's prayer followed by the song *Avinu Malkeinu*, by Barbra Streisand.

Chuck Miville gave the final sermon talking about why the Lord called Moose home on Father's Day. The microphone was then open for anyone who cared to say something. Barry spoke about what a blessing it had been to care for Moose. He was very emotional. Maria, her aide, told a story about how she had asked Moose to be a surrogate mother to her since she lived so far away from her own mother, to which Moose responded, "I'll try." She told sweet stories and read a poem. She later shared how frightened she was because she had never spoken publicly before. Peggy, the nurse, spoke about how great it was when she'd stop off to see how Moose was doing – and she would be out with us. She said she knew Moose was a part of life (instead of just waiting to die).

She also told a story about how Moose told her one day that she was a "damned fool" because she was being overly solicitous. Ron Coffin, the head of Hospice, spoke about Alzheimer's and how many seniors were suffering from the disease today and the decisions families will be forced to make. The service lasted two hours, but the time seemed to fly by for me.

Afterward, everyone enjoyed the deli trays, fresh fruit platters, coffee cakes, pastries, etc. People spilled out everywhere. I was relieved it was over. I believe Moose stuck around and was pleased with her memorial service. There was a rare blend of people at the house that day; Soldiers for Jesus, the owners of the Vietnamese restaurant, where Moose loved to eat (they would never charge for her meals) – Jew and Gentile alike came to honor her. I trust God that he answered our prayers for Moose's salvation, but there was no positive proof from her. That is why I wanted to cover the bases and honor her Jewish heritage, as well as, address and give the message of salvation. I wanted the Holy Spirit to conduct the service, so I didn't impose any restrictions on what was said.

I was concerned about Max. This was his first up-close-and-personal experience with death, other than a family pet. He was reluctant to discuss his feelings and left the service before it concluded. To this day, he does not want to be questioned about his feelings. He frequently talks about how much he misses his grandmother. Thank God all the negativity, associated with caring for her, evaporated and he is left with fond memories.

Our friend, Barbara, arrived late. She had lost her mother to the disease several years ago. Cheryl, Barry,

Barb and I plopped on the couch and watched the video of the funeral. Unfortunately, the battery gave out, but the mood of the day was captured.

In the following days, I busied myself with writing thank you notes and packing for our trip to visit Brandy and Dirk. I was looking forward to this vacation. It would be the first time we didn't need to call home checking on my mother. I was clear-headed – nothing to consider but having a relaxing time with my children and husband. I gave myself permission to sleep-in and indulge myself however, and whenever, I needed to. It was okay to be selfish with no guilt. I had completed my duty – seen it through to the end, with no regrets or second-guessing on whether I could've done things differently. It was time to enjoy life again and I was ready to jump in feet first.

Chapter XXVI

THE ASHES

My mother had specified her desire to be cremated while she was still lucid, years before her death. She had also told her sister, Lucille, of her desire and I assumed she had talked to Reuben because she would laughingly say, "Can you believe it? Reuben wants my ashes." I had preselected the mortuary and spoken with them about what was to be done.

There was no anguish over it when the time came. When I went to sign the authorization papers for cremation, I was told they would need Reuben's signature also.

I never expected any problems with this as I thought she made her wishes clear to everyone. We were at a florist, picking out flowers for the memorial service, when Barry received word that Reuben was resisting. He had refused to authorize cremation. Reuben and my nephew, Todd, wanted Moose's body shipped back to Chicago for burial next to my dad. I thought this was odd since nobody ever bothered to visit my father's gravesite, which had been duly noted by Moose.

We were all very upset. I wanted to honor my mother's wishes but the mortuary could not proceed unless both siblings agreed. Everyone tried to intercede, from the social worker to the conservator. I told them to call my aunt and verify if my mother had ever discussed her wishes with her. After a flurry of phone calls, Reuben conceded to cremation.

With this resolved, I could plan the funeral. I kept inquiring of the funeral director if he had heard from Reuben regarding the distribution of the cremains. He hadn't heard. Finally, I asked Kenny, the conservator, to ask Reuben what he wanted to do with the ashes. That was Friday night, the service was Sunday and we were leaving town to visit Brandy and Dirk the following Wednesday. I instructed the mortuary to take a small amount of ash out and place it in an urn for me. The remainder would be mailed to Reuben. I asked the director to please seal the urn so no ash could spill out. Tuesday, Kenny called saying that Reuben wanted all the ashes or none. I agreed and quickly called the mortuary to see if they could unseal the urn and place all the ashes in the box set aside for Reuben. They worked on the urn all day with a desolvant to no avail. Who could've known this would be a stumbling block?

When it was apparent that the urn could not be opened, I called Kenny to inform him of the situation, so he could call Reuben. This was not a malicious act. Rick said Kenny may have to get a court order to determine the fate of the ashes.

I said to Barry, "Reuben would never feel that he had gotten all the ashes no matter what happened." I didn't want ash issues robbing me of my peace.

After a long time, Kenny called back and said Reuben wouldn't feel comfortable that he had received all the ashes so we could keep them – an answer to prayer.

Chapter XXVII

THE RING

Nearly one month to the day of Moose's death, we received a request from Reuben, via Kenny, asking about a diamond initial ring. I told Kenny that my mother had given the ring to my son for his Bar Mitzvah since the diamond (MR) matched my son's initials, Maxwell Royce. I told him I'd be willing to give him another of my mother's rings – a jade, surrounded by diamonds, that my grandmother had designed for Moose.

I also said I would send back any of his family's pictures that Moose had in her possession. Against my husband's wishes, I sent off the package. Barry felt Reuben deserved nothing because he had made no attempts to see his mother the past three years. I felt maybe God was working on Reuben and he realized he had no momentos from either parent. Reuben didn't seem particularly interested in valued possessions handed down from generation to generation. I had collected, framed, and hung family pictures on my wall. I saved letters, jewelry, furniture, clothing, etc. Reuben and Sheryl, his wife, didn't seem to value anything my parents had offered them. They had received money, loans for businesses, etc, but not much in the way of memorabilia – their choice. When it was all over, the money spent, they had nothing to remind them of our parents.

The one thing that Reuben had received upon my grandmother's death was an autograph book with signatures from Ronald Reagan, Clark Gable, Gloria Swanson, and Elizabeth Taylor, left over from my grandmother's exclusive jewelry shop at the Ambassador East Hotel. I used to love looking over those signatures, but they went to my brother who auctioned them off for $1,200. I felt maybe he genuinely regretted the fact that he had nothing from my mother. I carefully packed up his family photos, the ring, and a picture of my mother when she became engaged to my father, along with a photo taken in a nightclub with aunts and uncles in the 1940s. I also selected, after much thought, a recent photo of my mother in a wheelchair. I hope, at last, he will value these things. It's between him and God if he sells the ring. It is his last opportunity to have something of hers.

Later, a message on the recorder from Kenny, stated that the package had arrived and Reuben was very, very happy with it.

My prayer is that one day Reuben and I can reconcile and reunite our families. I have forgiven him and fantasize that he reads this book and forgives and understands our action. At this time, I don't feel the door has been opened.

Chapter XXVIII

MOOSEHAVEN

Several days after my mother's memorial service, we began our new life without her, resuming our quest for a lakefront home. Max, Barry and I boarded a plane for Minnesota to visit our daughter and son-in-law. First, and foremost, I needed a rest. Secondarily, we were to search the state of "ten thousand lakes" for a new home.

I felt strangely irresponsible. The urge to call home to check on Moose's condition wasn't there. I had been released, emotionally, from my duties. While life returned to a comfortable normalcy, there was a hole in my spirit that Moose used to occupy. In contrast to the beginning of our journey to take care of Moose, the adjustment to be less responsible would no doubt be much easier. As our visit was coming to an end, it became apparent that finding just the right property, to serve as a family retreat, may still be out of reach. The day before we were to return home, our children remembered a resort area only 40 miles from their home in Moorhead. In one last desperate attempt, we phoned our realtor to meet us there and schedule some appointments. We eagerly packed into the car and headed out to our rendezvous point. On the way, serendipity came into play and we literally fell upon the property we'd been dreaming of. The sign on the road indicated that the property behind the dense trees, was for sale.

My son-in-law impulsively turned into the driveway, which wound it's way through a forest of oak, maple and spruce trees. A wood-carved plaque posted on one of the trees read, "Welcome To The Lake." Slowly, as we meandered through the vegetation, a small home appeared. A woman, the apparent owner, stepped out on the front porch.

"Can I help you?" she queried.

"Is this property still available?" my son-in-law asked. Sensing this could be the dream home we had been searching for diligently, since my husband had retired four years earlier, we all held our breath, until she responded, "yes."

Boldly, Dirk continued, "Can we see your home?" This was not the typical way one gained entrance to view a property, without an appointment. Nevertheless, we were willing to cast protocol aside to get our dream.

"No, I'm not prepared for a showing, but you can call my agent for an appointment," she answered.

"Well, you see," he continued undaunted, "my in-laws will be in town only one more day before returning to Colorado. Can we walk the grounds and look around?"

"Sure, suit yourselves," she responded.

The six of us scattered out of the car like roaches when the light is turned on. The land was expansive with rolling hills decorated with hundreds of mature trees. You couldn't see the road through all of the beautiful trees. But what took my breath away, was the magnificent view of the huge lake spread out beneath the bluff like a lush blue carpet. I knew, right then, this was to be our home. I didn't even care what the house looked like inside. The land captured my heart and imagination.

We walked down the gently sloping land to the dock. To the left, there was an ice-fishing hut pulled up on shore waiting for the winter. We swarmed all over the property, whispering, to camouflage our excitement. The other side of the house there was a fenced-in garden with a wood-carved sign above the gate, that read, "Garden of Eaten," that was equally captivating. Wild lilies bordered the fence enclosing the vegetable garden, laden with sugar peas, squash, peppers, tomatoes, lettuce and spinach. My imagination went wild, picturing myself on hands and knees in a straw hat planting in the spring. I was smitten. Beside the garden, was a bench carved from a tree stump. It was there I could rest and contemplate what I'd be planting. Also, beside the garden, was a grove of wild raspberry bushes. Brandy was sampling the fruit. I looked over and said, "Leave some for the owners, will you?" She giggled.

Elaborate bird houses were part of the natural landscape and the sweet sound of birds feasting and calling to one another, in stereo, provided the background music.

Jutting out from the back of the house was a large deck with built-in seating and a tree poking up through the middle–carefully planned, I thought. I imagined having my first cup of coffee in the early morning out there, looking over "my" lake. I had now made it very personal. It was "my" lake, suddenly. I recognized the signs alright. It's not like I was unknowledgeable. I had been a real estate broker for 12 years and a sophisticated trader. I knew I was hooked.

Once again, Dirk took command, knocking on the front door. The owner politely stepped out on the front porch. He asked the price of the home and if it included all of the land we had surveyed. Satisfied with her answer, we returned to the car assured that this was to be our new home.

I took one last look around at the vast stretch of

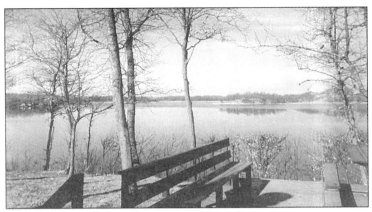
"Moose Haven" in the early spring.

water below before getting back into the car. Everything had come full cycle. I knew that this was my mother's gift to me. My family had interrupted pursuit of our lakefront home to care for Moose. It had been a three-year diversion that I was quite willing to take for her benefit. When things would get particularly tough, I remembered God's promise to me, "***Be patient and I will give you the desires of your heart.***" I whispered, "Thank you," before getting into the car.

We purchased that home for exactly the amount of money I received from my mother's estate. Moose has been laid to rest in a shady spot overlooking the lake, marked by a marble headstone reading, "Forever Dancing With The Angels," surrounded by beautiful flowers that we all planted.

But those who wait for the Lord shall change and renew their strength and power; they shall lift their wings and mount up as eagles; they shall run and not be weary, they shall walk and not faint or become tired. Isaiah 40:31

Chapter XXIX

POST SCRIPT BY DR. BARRY KRAFT:
The Psychological Impact of Alzheimer's on the Family

As a practicing psychiatrist for over twenty years, I had treated many people with dementia. I would hospitalize these patients when they became out of control and too difficult for their families to manage at home. During their hospital stay, I would stabilize them and arrange placement for them outside of the home. In retrospect, I had no understanding of what the patient or their family were really experiencing. The devastation to both parties is beyond comprehension unless you've experienced it yourself.

I have since repented for my lack of feeling and understanding and pray that this book, chronicling the journey with my mother-in-law, may be beneficial to those currently walking through the fire with their loved ones.

As Jewish Believers in Christ as the Messiah, we believed God called us to honor Moose, both as Fran's mother and as a widow. This mission came unexpectedly, at a time when I had retired from a very active practice and for the first time in my life had the finances and freedom to do what I wanted.

I must admit to feeling angry at times because I'd been able to retire at a relatively young age and was looking forward to the fruits of all my work. Having

Moose live with us was like living at the hospital 24 hours a day, instead of the normal 12-15 hours I put in during my practice. I was used to being awakened several times at night when I was on call, but having the monitor on was like being on call constantly. We suffered from persistent sleep deprivation. It has been two years since Moose's death and we are just now recovering.

Even though we had ample help, our day was very fragmented. It was difficult to carve out enough time for just ourselves. We would anxiously await the arrival of an aide so we could grab a few hours to take in dinner and a movie. We were so tightly scheduled, that if someone arrived late, it would throw off our entire evening. When we did manage to break away, any positive effect was instantly erased as our car re-entered the driveway. As caregivers, the responsibility hung over our head like a huge black cloud that never goes away. Knowing we were returning to our duties, never fully allowed us to relax while we are away.

The amount of energy required both physically and emotionally left us drained. It effects things like sexual desire and the ability to emotionally give to others besides the patient. We were still the parents of two children who needed us as well.

In addition to being involved parents, we had been mentors to many in our community. The strength to continue in this capacity came only from God. We felt totally depleted of our own resources and were completely dependent on the Lord.

Given the hardships we had to endure, the many wonderful, heartwarming moments more than compensated us. In subsequent conversations we've had with our children, none of us would exchange the price we had to pay for the rewards we have reaped here on earth. We have no regrets about how we handled the situation. We felt that we answered the call to duty.

Many times God chooses the least likely person to carry out His tasks. Often it is not the favored child or the child who is emotionally closest to the parent who becomes the designated caregiver. This is a double-edged sword because, on one hand, there is a natural resentment for the least favored having to take on the tremendous burden of care. On the other hand, it gives the caregiver the chance to work through issues that would never have been resolved without the close contact. This was the case with Fran and her mother. The hidden blessing in caring for Moose, was that it allowed Fran to address life-long issues that hindered their relationship. When Moose finally went "home," there was no lingering anger or guilt on Fran's part. She was able to peacefully walk Moose to heaven's gate. It was an interesting process watching Fran deal with conflicting feelings toward her mother. She vacillated between feelings of frustration and joy as Moose was able to show her softer side. As the disease progressed, Moose became child-like, sweet and even expressed gratitude for what we were doing. Ironically, the three years we spent caring for Moose, were the best of their entire relationship. I watched as the disease took its toll on both Fran and Moose. Fran was always tired, stressed and continually grieving as each of Moose's functions faded away.

A reversal of roles slowly evolved. Fran was protective of her mother. Especially, when Moose was living on her own. Fran tried to insure that her mother's dignity remained intact and that she wouldn't be rejected by other residents at the assisted-care living facility. But

Moose had her own survival instincts by gravitating to people on her level. The ultimate reversal of roles began when Moose resorted to calling Fran, "Mother." As she regressed, an intense sibling rivalry between Moose and our children developed. Thank God, for our children's understanding of the situation and the grace they were able to show Moose.

Even though, at the end, Moose was completely dependent on others, she had a nobility about her like never before. As her ability to speak waned, we tried hard to remember that there was still a human being with real emotions, imprisoned in her body. We spoke to her, not about her as if she were invisible. Without words, she developed an ability to communicate through facial expressions. With a glance, she could speak volumes.

Fran instructed all the caretakers that her mother was to be well-groomed daily and treated respectfully. She was a valued member of our family and we included her in our activities. Because we respected her, our friends and our children's friends did likewise. Amazingly, until the day she died, she was able to form new relationships which we encouraged. Our home was open at all times for people to drop in for a visit with her. As it became more difficult for us to get out, we brought life into the house. We strived to provide a stimulating atmosphere for her to thrive in.

Our son, Max, was 14 when Moose came to live with us. At a time when teenagers are most vulnerable and concerned about what their peers think about them and their families, Max was in the trenches caring for his ailing grandmother. He helped Fran with her toileting procedures and carried her in and out of the car. His courage and strength were remarkable.

Because of the sibling rivalry, he was often the target of her anger and frustration. She would strike out at him, trying to scratch and hit him as he lifted her into bed or onto the portable toilet. He was the most challenged because of his age. We didn't soften the experience for him. He had a firsthand glimpse at the finality of death and didn't flinch.

In a paper Max wrote for school, he described the disease as "a personality altering process. I remember Moose as getting very aggressive and then becoming docile and child-like. I liked her best when our roles had reversed and I became her caretaker." He further stated, "It is really hard to deal with the hurt, anger, rage etc. that you can experience when taking care of someone with the disease. Often the person can be verbally, mentally and physically abusive to the caregivers. They can break into sudden fits of rage in which they will pinch, kick, bite, punch, claw and scream at you. This is not because they are evil people, it's just one of the horrible side effects of this dreaded disease. My grandmother would attack at least one of us every single day."

Even exposed to Alzheimer's at its worst, Max viewed the experience as enriching by saying, "Her life was valuable because she taught us more about patience and unconditional love than any other human being. She became our teacher and my love for her grew greatly while she was in our care."

In recollecting his experience now, he fondly talks about his grandmother, illustrating that when you get to the other side of it, the essence remaining is sweet. Because of how well he handled the situation, he has earned our respect and proven himself to be a man of substance at a very young age. Our goal was to model for our children how they are to honor their parents. People are not disposable when they develop problems.

Max has learned a life lesson that no school can ever teach. Both of our children were enlightened by having their grandmother live with us. We had never lived near relatives before, and although Moose's life was somewhat impaired because of her condition, it was wonderful having her around. The first year she was with us, we tried to make it as normal as possible, taking her to the movies, theater, restaurants, ballet, etc. When she was initially hospitalized for diagnosis, she would see the children, not us. There had developed a bond between them.

Our daughter, Brandy, had more of a life outside the home. She was a graduating senior in college and had become engaged during this period. She had more diversions than Max. She struggled with guilt because she wanted to be more helpful but her involvements took her attention elsewhere. I remember a conversation with Fran when our daughter went to visit her fiance for two weeks. Fran felt jealous that Brandy could be more carefree, while it was definitely Fran's turn to be responsible, stepping up to bat to care for her mother.

The wedding festivities were a great diversion for all of us, including Moose. We kept her informed and involved in all of the wedding activities. Brandy's future in-laws always included Moose in their invitations for holiday dinners. Moose was always part of the equation. The wedding kept her focused on a future event.

Again as a result of sibling rivalry, Brandy was often the object of Moose's anger and jealousy, even to the point where she demanded to wear white, thinking she was the bride. She would scowl at Brandy every time Brandy would enter the room. Brandy had a difficult time understanding why she was on the receiving end of Moose's wrath. I know it was taxing for Brandy, sharing her mother's attention, while she was preparing to be married. To Brandy's credit, at no time did she hide her grandmother in fear that somehow her wedding would be disrupted by Moose's behavior. Moose was able to attend both Brandy's graduation and wedding without incident.

Some helpful hints that we can impart are:

1. Keep your loved one involved in family activities.

2. Because of our attitude, friends embraced Moose, including her in invitations.

3. We would get her out of the house every day. She loved going for rides. We kept seeking places to take her i.e. malls, food courts.

4. We found restaurants that honored the elderly and welcomed us. We would take her there at off hours when they weren't real crowded.

5. We talked to her and didn't treat her like less of a person because she couldn't talk.

6. We took her to performances of Barry and Max's band, who always dedicated a song to her.

7. We took her to church, until she became too disruptive and then we formed a home church.

8. When it became difficult to take her out, we brought social life into the home, i.e. pot luck dinners,

Scrabble® nights with friends and home movies.

9. We always acted as her advocate, trying new ways to approach a problem.

10. We kept her well groomed, so she always looked nice.

11. We didn't make her feel bad about being incontinent.

12. We honored her wishes as we understood them.

13. We had the courts appoint a conservator when she showed inability to manage her own financial affairs. We kept ourselves above reproach.

14. Although she had no concept of money, she received an allowance. We would instruct aides to take her to lunch and have her pay her own way.

15. We embraced her as part of the family, until she died.

16. We didn't let the illness be an excuse for bad behavior.

17. We never gave up hope. We would keep trying different things for her memory.

18. We tried to soften the blow over each lost skill.

19. It is important to discuss your feelings among the family members.

20. We availed ourselves to counselling, provided by Hospice.

21. We sought the counsel of others who had gone

through similar experiences and in turn, shared information with others. Networking is invaluable.

22. Seek reliable sources for in-home caretakers. Ask for references when hiring. If necessary, set up surveillance to make sure your loved one is well cared for in your absence.

23. It is important to remember as caretaker – you may also still be a wife, mother, etc., to others. Take a break once in a while.

24. Don't feel guilty if you can't be a direct caregiver – it's not for everybody.

25. Stay on top of medical problems as they develop.

26. Pray and seek prayer from others. Let those around you lend support.

27. We loved Moose unconditionally, as Jesus loves us.

Our prayer for this book is that perhaps, something we did to enhance Moose's last years will help those of you currently struggling with a loved one suffering from Alzheimer's. To ensure that any questions you may have will be answered, you may call us at our home, 218-863-2469. God bless each of you.

Chapter XXX

POST SCRIPT BY DR. BETH M. LEY:

Nutritional and Supplemental Considerations for the Treatment and Prevention of Alzheimer's and Dementia

At birth, the human brain contains as many as one hundred billion nerve cells. From then on there is a continuous process of decline. Brain weight decreases gradually over time – about 10% over a normal life span, due to neuron death.

Different parts of the brain lose neurons at different rates. In most brain stem regions below the cerebral cortex (the area responsible for automatic unlearned activity (breathing, heart pumping, blinking, etc.), there is little or no cell loss with advancing age. In comparison, the cerebral cortex, which is responsible for thinking and memory, loses up to 50,000 neurons a day.

The hippocampus is the specific region of the brain known to be important for memory. New hippocampus cells continually replace old ones. Numerous factors determine the rate at which this is done. Factors which affect overall mental functioning include:

✧ Optimal nutrition.

✧ Optimal circulation to the brain bringing oxygen, glucose and nutrients.

✧ Oxidative stress (exposure to free radicals).

✧ Mental and physical stress and other factors which effect cortisol (a stress hormone) levels.

✧ Exposure to alcohol and certain drugs (both recreational and pharmaceutical).

✧ Environmental stimuli, (i.e. education).

✧ Genetics.

More common than actual cell death is the loss of the connections between neurons. With aging, dendritic branching of the individual nerve cells decreases, reducing the number of connections between neurons.

Alzheimer's disease (AD), a form of senile dementia, is a progressive and degenerative neurological disorder that results in memory impairment, as well as deterioration in cognitive function, reasoning, and behavior. It is the most common form of dementia, accounting for more than 60% of late-life cognitive dysfunction.

The loss of intellectual function caused by this disease, interferes with daily life and the ability to remain independent is soon lost. The condition may last many years, often eventually resulting in death due to factors such as compromised nutrition, complications of the immune system (i.e., pneumonia, sepsis, other infections), trauma, or aspiration.

The Signs of AD: Neuronal destruction that manifests as cortical atrophy, degeneration of the cholinergic neurons, and accumulation of neuritic plaques and neurofibrillary tangles occurs in the brains of individuals with Alzheimer's disease. A specific protein, beta amyloid, is found at the center of these neuritic plaques.

Other factors include concentrations of apolipoprotein E, inflammatory mediators such as prostaglandins, and the degree of cholinergic neuronal activity. Also, hormonal fluctuations may influence the condition's process, as demonstrated by a protective effect of estrogen observed in some studies.

AD begins with almost imperceptible changes. As the disease progresses, gradual memory loss, a decline in performance of routine tasks, increasing disorientation, impaired judgment, mood swings, personality changes, difficulty in learning, and a loss of language skills can occur. The progression of these manifestations demonstrates a high degree of variability, with courses lasting from 3 years to 20 years. Average survival after diagnosis is between 4 and 8 years.

Natural Support

Basic body functions such as nutritional and immune system status are affected negatively during the natural aging process. In Alzheimer's disease, there is an acceleration in the decline of these basic functions.

The dietary supplements discussed here (readily found in most health food stores or alternative care physicians' offices) may be beneficial in supporting Alzheimer's patients as well as decreasing the symptoms, rate of decline, and reducing the incidence of this disease.

Acetyl-L-Carnitine (ALC)

ALC is an important transport molecule in mitochondrial energy production. Enhanced activity of this molecule may be beneficial in the preservation and enhancement of neuronal function.

ALC, reportedly, can improve cellular oxygenation and prevent damage to cells. It also can facilitate and enhance the activity of cholinergic and dopaminergic neurons in the central nervous system. Additionally, it can increase synthesis of nerve growth factors as well as the expression of receptors for this hormone.

ALC is synthesized normally in the human body. While no specific symptoms have been identified with ALC deficiency, relative deficiency of this transport molecule could result in decreased energy production and age-related cognitive decline.

Dosage: 500-2,000 mg. daily in divided doses. Occasionally, side effects of mild abdominal discomfort, restlessness, vertigo, and headache have been reported.

Alpha-GPC (Alpha-Glycerylphosphorylcholine)

This is a derivative of soy lecithin that contains the essential nutrient choline. Alpha-GPC serves as a direct precursor in the synthesis of choline in the body.

Choline is a precursor of the important neurotransmitter, acetylcholine. Choline supplementation increases the level of acetylcholine in the memory circuits of the temporal lobe of the brain. Acetylcholine-sensitive neurons serve many different functions in the brain including the control of arousal, learning, motor activity and deep sleep, known as Rapid Eye Movement (REM) sleep.

Studies conducted at the National Institutes of Health showed that choline supplementation improves learning and memory in both normal individuals and in individuals with AD. (Sitaram) It has also shown to enhance memory in young individuals.

In addition to its brain enhancing benefits, increased choline may also enhance Growth Hormone (GH) release. This effect may be even more pronounced in older individuals who may have depressed levels. GH levels significantly decline with age. The decline of GH is related to many symptoms of aging such as muscle atrophy, decreased energy and sexual function, increased body fat, increased risk of cardiovascular disease, osteoporosis, and wrinkles. Clinical evidence suggests that by replacing GH, many of these symptoms can be reversed. Animal and human studies have demonstrated that

Alpha-GPC stimulates the secretion of GH from the pituitary, making this supplement in high demand by all those concerned about aging! (Ghigo, Ceda)

Alpha-GPC may be useful to help reduce some of the neurological decline that occurs with aging as it has demonstrated significant beneficial effects upon cognitive function, memory impairments and dementia. (Frattola, Muratorio, Abbati, Di Perri)

Supplementing Alpha-GPC is preferred over supplementing choline or lecithin because Alpha-GPC allows for larger amounts of choline to be absorbed into the intestinal tract. (Zeisel)

Dosage: 100-500 mg. daily

α–Lipoic Acid (Alpha Lipoic Acid)

α–Lipoic Acid is a powerful antioxidant that works synergistically with Vitamins C and E and glutathione, and helps regenerate C and E for re-use. It also supports the proper functioning of two key enzymes that convert food into energy.

The brain is subject to antioxidant stress just like the rest of the body. Antioxidant stress can contribute to circulatory problems and damage to brain cells. α–Lipoic Acid aids brain wellness because of its ability to neutralize potentially toxic substances and oxidants. (Siesjd, McCord)

The higher the level of antioxidants and the longer we can keep these antioxidants regenerating, the longer we are protected from oxidative damage. As antioxidant levels diminish, our vulnerability to neurological damage increases.

Animal studies have shown that α–Lipoic Acid is beneficial in helping to restore lost memory in aging subjects, but does not improve memory beyond what is normal in young healthy individuals. In mice, α–Lipoic Acid improved performance in an open-field memory test. The α–Lipoic Acid-treated animals actually performed slightly better than young animals, 24 hours after the first test. The authors concluded that α–Lipoic Acid's free radical scavenging ability may improve N-methyl-o-aspartate receptor density, which leads to improved memory in older individuals. (Stoll)

The oxidative-stress hypothesis, as a cause of Alzheimer's, encourages antioxidant use for prevention and therapy. The toxicity of amyloid beta-protein, an amino acid peptide associated with plaques in the brains of Alzheimer's patients, seems also to be due to oxidative stress in neurons, and also potential sources of free radicals in brain tissue. (Behl)

Several other studies also suggest that free radicals are involved in the pathogenesis of AD, and that antioxidant nutrients may be very useful in prevention. (Evans)

Dosage: 50-400 mg. daily

Ashwagandha

This ancient Indian herb helps relieve stress, and is traditionally used for enhancement of memory, learning and sex drive. It promotes relaxation when sleep is desired, by soothing the nerves and restoring strength. This herb may help reduce levels of elevated cortisol (often referred to as the stress hormone). Elevated cortisol levels are known to have a detrimental effect on memory by interfering with cell regeneration in the hippocampus region of the brain. (Suemaru, Newcomer)

It also has antioxidant properties, which may explain some of its pharmacological effects. (Panda)

Dosage: 100-200 mg. daily

Bacopa (Bacopa monniera)

Bacopa monniera is an Ayurvedic botanical with apparent anti-anxiety, anti-fatigue, and memory-strengthening effects. It has been used historically for restoring cognitive function. (Kidd) It is well known as an adaptogen and a brain tonic for improving the intellect, memory and increasing longevity.

Bacopa strengthens the veins and capillaries, increasing circulation and delivery of oxygen and nutrients. Bacopa helps alleviate fatigue and promotes relaxation when sleep is desired. In addition to increasing brain function, it may also increase sex drive.

The botanical's saponin compounds (bacosides) are alleged to have the capability to enhance nerve impulse transmission and thereby strengthen memory and general cognition. Clinically, bacopa has been reported to be a useful agent for improving intellectual behavior in children and to reduce anxiety in adults. It is one of the most popular supplements used in India for mental disorders and anxiety neurosis. (Singh, R.H.)

Dosage: 50-150 mg. taken 3 times a day and standardized to contain at least 20% bacosides A and B per dose. While reported to be safe in these dosages, it should be used with caution in individuals taking calcium channel blocking agents.

Colostrum

This immune-enhancing supplement is largely used to boost overall resistance to disease and infection, but anecdotal reports also claim improvement in memory and mental functioning in individuals in the early stages of dementia and AD.

Dosage: 1 150-200 mg. lozenge 3-4 times daily or 1 ml. liquid administered sublingually.

CoQ10 (Coenzyme Q10)

The brain tissue contains a high level of CoQ10 suggesting the potential usefulness of supplemental CoQ10 in the treatment of neuro-degenerative diseases.

The Proceeding of the National Academy of Sciences reports that CoQ10 supplementation, which increases concentrations of brain mitochondria (which produce energy), is neuroprotective. COQ10 levels are markedly decreased in damaged cells produced by administration of a known toxic substance.

In a study at Massachusetts General Hospital and Harvard Medical School, Boston, MA, oral administration of CoQ10 in 12-month-old rats, resulted in significant increases in CoQ10 in the mitochondria in the cerebral cortex. The CoQ10 also significantly increased the life span of the animals. (Matthews)

Individuals with AD have depressed CoQ10. (Edlund) While studies show that antioxidants such as Vitamin E are neuroprotective in individuals with Alzheimer's, there are no published studies involving supplemental CoQ10 and this degenerative condition.

Dosage: 200 mg. daily. High CoQ10 doses (600-1,200 mg. daily) have been used in some of the studies involving Parkinson's and Huntington's diseases to obtain beneficial results. These dosage levels were found to be safe and effective with only mild side effects. (Feigin, Schultz)

DHA (Docosahexaenoic Acid)

DHA is an essential fatty acid (EFA), meaning it is an essential part of our daily diet. It is a member of the Omega-3 family, and is the longest of the long-chain polyunsaturated fatty acids (22:6n-3). It is the most sensitive to destruction and damage (mostly due to free radicals) both inside and outside the body. DHA is commonly deficient in the diet and body.

DHA: The Most Abundant Structural Fat in the Brain! DHA is of critical importance as it is the basic building block of each cell formed. Brain tissue is about 60% structural fat, of which about 25% is DHA. Brain and other nervous tissues are unique in containing this high concentration of DHA.

Each of the fourteen billion cells which make up the grey matter of the brain has connecting arms ending in synapses. These electrical currents between brain cells, send messages throughout the body. When the arms are intact, communication is efficient. If the arms harden due to aging or free radical damage, signal transmission slows and may be altered. Adequate DHA helps keep the connections functional. Low levels can cause connections to lose efficiency, leading to brain and memory disorders.

Studies suggest that DHA supplementation may be helpful for the elderly, who require high levels of brain nutrients. Dr. Ernst Schaefer, of the Human Nutrition Center on Aging at Tufts University, reports that a low level of DHA is a significant risk factor for dementia – almost twice the risk of developing dementia over the next nine years than with those whose blood levels of DHA were high. (Schaefer)

In a Japanese study, patients taking 700-1,400 mg. of DHA daily, showed a large improvement in dementia (cooperation, speech, depression, and other psychological symptoms). The study found that the dementia in 69% of those individuals was due to blood vessel problems. (Yazawa)

Alzheimer's Patients Have DHA Deficiency. Recent developments show that the brains of individuals who have died from Alzheimer's, have an EFA deficiency, particularly DHA. Studies show that patients with Alzheimer's who receive EFA plus antioxidants show improvement consistently better than those not receiving fatty acids. (Corrigan)

Faulty brain cell membranes are also associated with the increased release of beta amyloid proteins. Beta amyloid proteins appear to be the principal active constituent of senile plaques thought to be a probable cause of brain damage, resulting in Alzheimer's. (Newman)

DHA and other fatty acids are at high risk for oxidation in the brain, contributing to increased degradation of brain phospholipids in Alzheimer's disease. This was demonstrated by significantly decreased brain levels of membrane DHA and other fatty acids in Alzheimer's patients compared to controls. (Prasad)

This reinforces the importance of protective antioxidants such a Vitamins C and E, lipoic acid, ginkgo biloba, etc., which help prevent oxidative damage in the brain and throughout the body.

Dosage: 3,000-8,000 mg. (DHA/EPA combo) daily. The uptake of fatty acids into the neuronal tissue can be very slow and it may take six to eight months or longer to see changes in the brain and other nervous tissue. Many degenerative conditions do not develop "overnight" and cannot be expected to be reversed quickly either.

Ginkgo Biloba

This botanical has been used extensively as a medicinal agent worldwide for centuries. Its main active components are the flavoglycosides. These compounds act as free radical scavengers or antioxidants. Ginkgo biloba reportedly improves circulation in the elderly, which can lead to enhanced memory and delayed onset of AD as well as reductions of senile dementia, tinnitus, and vertigo. The herb's memory-enhancing effects, reportedly, can benefit younger individuals as well.

In addition, ginkgo biloba can inhibit platelet-activating factor (PAF), which can possibly reduce the adhesive nature of platelets. (Braquet) The plant may increase cerebral brain flow as well, enhancing the delivery of nutrients to the brain and enhancing the elimination of cell metabolism byproducts and oxygenating the tissues.

Ginkgo biloba also may normalize acetylcholine (ACh) receptors and improve cholinergic function, which is important in Alzheimer's patients, as well as improve glucose utilization in brain cells. (Ramassamy)

Dosage: 40-80 mg. of standardized extract, 3 times daily. Extract should be standardized to 24% ginkgo biloba flavoglycosides and 6% triterpenes per dose. It also may be standardized to 27/7 or 32/9 per dose.

Ginkgo biloba is generally safe and side effects from it are rare. The most typical side effects of this botanical are gastrointestinal distress, headache, and allergic skin reactions. (Odawara) Ginkgo biloba should be used with caution when taken with the following medications:

1. Anticoagulants – due to PAF inhibition.

2. Aspirin or nonsteroidal anti-inflammatory drugs (NSAIDs) – may increase GI bleeding.

3. Monoamine oxidase (MAO) inhibitors – may enhance the effects of these medications.

Huperzine A

This botanical constituent is derived from Chinese club moss (Huperzia serrata), which has been used for centuries to treat various health problems, including memory and alertness-related conditions.

Huperzine A is currently used as an acetylcholinesterase (AchE) inhibitor in senile dementia and Alzheimer's disease. In the 1980s, scientists demonstrated that purified huperzine A can keep AchE from breaking down acetylcholine. Huperzine seems to protect the AchE from interacting with the soman nerve agent, which is subsequently metabolized and inactivated in the body.

Dosage: 50 mcg. taken 1-3 times daily. This natural medicine is reported safe in recommended dosages. However, based on pharmacology, it should be used with caution in combination with anticholinergic agents.

Phosphatidylserine (PS)

PS belongs to the class of fat-soluble compounds called phospholipids. Phospholipids are essential cell membrane components that are found in very high concentrations within the brain. PS actually is the most abundant phospholipid found in brain tissue.

PS helps provide cellular membranes with their fluidity, flexibility, and permeability. It stimulates the release of various neurotransmitters, such as acetylcholine and dopamine. Also, it enhances ion transport and increases the number of certain neurotransinitter receptor sites in the brain. The symptoms of PS deficiency include depression, memory loss, and cognitive decline.

Dosage: 100 mg. taken 1-3 times daily. It is reportedly very safe in recommended dosages.

Vinpocetine

Vinpocetine is derived from vincamine, which is an extract of the lesser periwinkle plant (Vinca minor). This botanical constituent increases metabolism in the brain in four ways:

• Increases blood flow.
• Increases the rate at which brain cells produce adenosine triphosphate (ATP).

- Speeds up the use of glucose in the brain.
- Speeds up the use of oxygen in the brain.

Vinpocetine is used as a cerebral metabolic enhancing agent for memory enhancement and increased brain function. Because of its stimulating effect on blood flow, this plant constituent also has been used to treat circulatory problems in the brain such as memory problems due to low circulation.

Dosage: 10-20 mg. twice daily. It is safe in recommended dosage.

Vitamin C (Mineral Ascorbates)

The brain is the second largest user of Vitamin C in the body. This should give you an idea of how important it is to help us think better and also to protect us, for example, to avoid stroke. Vitamin C is needed to produce many of the message carriers for the entire body, including serotonin, which is involved in appetite and sleep regulation.

Mineral ascorbates (such as calcium or magnesium ascorbate) is the form of C that the body actually uses. Other forms of C, such as ascorbic acid, must first be converted into mineral ascorbates (calcium ascorbate, potassium ascorbates, etc,) in order to be used.

Antioxidants, such as ascorbates, which have been shown to reduce oxidative damage, may be protective against poor memory, which is a major component of dementia disorders such as Parkinson's and Alzheimer's.

Vitamin C levels are depressed among individuals with Alzheimer's, even though their intake of C-containing foods is similar to individuals without Alzheimer's disease. (Riviere) At least one study has demonstrated the reduced incidence of Alzheimer's among individuals 65 years and older, who supplement Vitamin C. (Morris)

Numerous studies suggest that Vitamin C protects against cognitive impairment. (Paleologos, Lonnrat) As a powerful antioxidant, ascorbate is protective of the neural tissues that are at risk of free radical damage.

Dosage: 2,000-8,000 mg. daily

Vitamin E

There is much written about the important antioxidant protective properties of Vitamin E. Recently, Vitamin E has demonstrated its ability to prevent learning and memory deficits caused by amyloid beta-peptide, the major constituent of the senile plaques in the brains of patients with Alzheimer's. (Yamada)

Dosage: 600-1,200 IU daily

Zinc

This important mineral is required for protein synthesis and collagen formation. It promotes a healthy immune system and protects the liver from chemical damage. Deficiency may result in memory impairment, fatigue, high cholesterol levels, impaired night vision, weakened immune system, slow or impaired wound healing, and a propensity toward diabetes, prostate trouble, or impotence. Stress tends to deplete zinc stores from the body.

Studies have shown that depleted zinc levels are very common in Alzheimer's patients. (Corrigan)

Dosage: 10-25 mg. daily

Note: This information is not intended as medical advice. Its purpose is solely educational. Please consult your healthcare professional for all health problems.

References

Alvarez XA; Laredo M; Corzo D; et al; Citicoline improves memory performance in elderly subjects. Methods Find Exp Clin Pharmacol 1997 Apr;19(3):201-10.

Barbiroli, B., Medori, R., Tritschler, H.J., et al: Lipoic (thioctic) acid increases brain energy availability and skeletal muscle performance as shown by in vivo 31P-MRS in a patient with mitochondrial cytopathy. J Neurol 1995 Jul;242(7):472-7.

Beal MF; Matthews RT; Coenzyme Q10 in the central nervous system and its potential usefulness in the treatment of neurodegenerative diseases. Massachusetts General Hospital, Boston Mol Aspects Med 1997: 18 Suppl:S169-7960.

Beal, MF, et al; Coenzyme Q10 and nicotinamide block striatal lesions produced by the mitochondrial toxin malonate, Annals of Neurology, 1994;36;882-8.

Behl C, Amyloid beta-protein toxicity and oxidative stress in Alzheimer's disease. Max Planck Institute of Psychiatry, Clinical Institute, Kraepelinstr. 2-10, D-80804 Munich, Germany. chris@mpipsykl.mpg.de Cell Tissue Res 1997 Dec;290(3):471-80

Behl C; Sagara YMechanism of amyloid beta protein induced neuronal cell death: current concepts and future perspectives. J Neural Transm Suppl 1997;49:125-34

Bhatti JZ; Hindmarch I; Vinpocetine effects on cognitive impairments produced by flunitrazepam. Int Clin Psychopharmacol 1987 Oct;2(4):325-31.

Blusztajn JK; Liscovitch M; Mauron C; et al; Phosphatidylcholine as a precursor of choline for acetylcholine synthesis. Neural Transm Suppl 1987;24:247-59.

Braquet, P; Anti-anaphylactic propertries of BN52021: A potent PAF antagonist, Adv Exp Med Biol 215-233, 1987.

Cameron HA; McKay R; Stem cells and neurogenesis in the adult brain. Laboratory of Molecular Biology, National Institutes of Health, Bethesda, Maryland Curr Opin Neurobiol 1998 Oct;8(5):677-80.

Cacabelos R; Caamano J; et al; Therapeutic effects of CDP-choline in Alzheimer's disease. Cognition, brain mapping, cerebrovascular hemodynamics, and immune factors. Institute for CNS Disorders, Basic and Clinical Neurosciences Research Center, La Coruna, Spain, Ann N Y Acad Sci 1996 Jan 17;777:399-403.

Ceda, G.P., et al; Effects pfCytidine5'Diphosphocholine administration on basal and GH releaseing secretion in elderly subjects, Acta Endocrinol. 1991. May; 124(5) 516-520.

Ceda, G.P., et al.; Alpha-GPC administration increases GH responses to GHRH of young and elderly sunjects. Horm. Metab. Res. 1992 Mar;24(3):119-121.

Corrigan FM; et al; EFAs in Alxheimer's Disease. Ann NY AcadAci, 1991;6640:250-2.

Corrigan FM; Reynolds GP; Ward NI; Hippocampal tin, aluminium and zinc in Alzheimer's disease. Argyll & Bute Hospital, Lochgilphead, UK. Biometals 1993 Autumn;6(3):149-54.

Corrigan FM; Mowat B; et al.; High density lipoprotein fatty acids in dementia. Argyll and Bute NHS Trust, Argyll and Bute Hospital, Lochgilphead, UK. Prostaglandins Leukot Essential Fatty Acids 1998 Feb;58(2):125-7.

Crook, T., et al; Effects of phosphatidylserine in Alzheimer's disease. Psychopharmacol Bull. 1992;28:61-6.

Edlund C; et al Ubiquinone, dolichol, and cholesterol metabolism in aging and Alzheimer's disease. Biochem Cell Biol 1992 Jun;70(6):422-8.

Eriksson PS; Perfilieva E; Bjork-Eriksson T; Alborn AM; Nordborg C; Peterson DA; Neurogenesis in the adult human hippocampus. Nat Med 1998 Nov;4(11):1313-7.

Evans DA; Morris MC, Is a randomized trial of antioxidants in the primary prevention of Alzheimer disease warranted? Alzheimer Dis Assoc Disord 1996 Fall;10 Suppl 1:45-9.

Gaal L; Molnar P; Effect of vinpocetine on noradrenergic neurons in rat locus coeruleus. Eur J Pharmacol 1990 Oct 23;187(3):537-9.

Ghigo, E, et al; Loe doses of either IV or orally administered arginine are able to enhance GH response to GHRHsecretion in elderly subjects, J. Endocrinol Invest. 1994, Feb;17(2):113-117.

Gotz ME, Dirr A, Gsell W, Burger R, Janetzky B, Freyberger A, Reichmann H, et al; Influence of N-methyl-4-phenyl-1,2,3,6-tetrahydropyridine, a-Lipoic Acid and L-deprenyl on the interplay between cellular redox systems. J Neural Transm Suppl 1994;43:145-62.

Grassel E Effect of Ginkgo-biloba extract on mental performance. Double-blind study using computerized measurement conditions in patients with cerebral insufficiency Fortschr Med 1992 Feb 20;110(5):73-6

Kidd PM; A review of nutrients and botanicals in the integrative management of cognitive dysfunction Contributing Editor, Alternative Medicine Review. Correspondence address:47 Elm St., El Cerrito, CA. Altern Med Rev 1999 Jun;4(3):144-61.

Kiss B; Karpati E; [Mechanism of action of vinpocetine] Vinpocetin hatasai, hatasmechanizmusa. Richter Gedeon Vegyeszeti Gyar Rt., Farmakologiai Kutato Kozpont, Budapest.Acta Pharm Hung 1996 Sep;66(5):213-24.

Koroshetz WJ; Jenkins BG; Rosen BR; Beal MF; Energy metabolism defects in Huntington's disease and effects of coenzyme Q10. Neurology Service, Mass. General Hospital and Harvard Medical School, Boston. Ann Neurol 1997; Feb;41(2):160-546.

Lakics V; Sebestyen MG; Erdo SL;Vinpocetine is a highly potent neuroprotectant against veratridine-induced cell death in primary cultures of rat cerebral cortex. CNS Pharmacology Lab, Budapest, Hungary. Neurosci Lett 1995 Feb 9;185(2):127-30.

Lonnrot K; Metsa-Ketela T; et al; *The effect of ascorbate and ubiquinone supplementation on plasma and CSF total antioxidant capacity.* Free Radic Biol Med 1996;21(2):211-7.

Maire JC; Wurtman RJ; Choline production from choline-containing phospholipids: a hypothetical role in Alzheimer's disease and aging. Prog Neuropsycho-pharmacol Biol Psychiatry 1984;8(4-6):637-42.

Miyazaki M; The effect of a cerebral vasodilator, vinpocetine, on cerebral vascular resistance evaluated by the Doppler ultrasonic technique in patients with cerebrovascular diseases. Department of Internal Medicine, Rohju Sanatorium, Osaka, Japan.Angiology 1995 Jan;46(1):53-8.

Miyata N; Yamaura H; Tanaka M; et al; Effects of VA-045, a novel apovincaminic acid derivative, on isolated blood vessels: cerebroarterial selectivity. Research Center, Taisho Pharmaceutical Co., Ltd., Saitama, Japan. Life Science

Monteleone P; Maj M; et al; Blunting by chronic phosphatidylserine administration of the stress- induced activation of the hypothalamo-pituitary-adrenal axis in healthy men. Institute of Psychiatry, University of Naples, Italy. Eur J Clin Pharmacol 1992;42(4):385-8.

Monteleone P; Beinat L; et al; Effects of phosphatidylserine on the neuroendocrine response to physical stress in humans. Institute of Medical Psychology and Psychiatry, First Medical School, University of Naples, Italy. Neuroendocrinology 1990 Sep;52(3):243-8.

Morris, MC; et al; Vitamin E and Vitamin C Supplement Use and Risk of Incident Alzheimer Disease, Alzheimer Disease and Associated Disorders; Vol 112; No 3, 121-126.

Newcomer JW; Selke G; Melson AK; et al;Decreased memory performance in healthy humans induced by stress-level cortisol treatment. Department of Psychiatry, Washington University School of Medicine, St Louis, MO. Arch Gen Psychiatry 1999 Jun;56(6):527-33.

Newman PE; Could diet be one of the causal factors of Alzheimer's disease? Source: Med Hypotheses, 1992 Oct, 39:2, 123-6.

Odawara M, et al. Ginkgo biloba, Neurology 48(3):789-790, 1997.

Orvisky E; Soltes L; Stancikova M; High-molecular-weight hyaluronan—a valuable tool in testing the antioxidative activity of amphiphilic drugs stobadine and vinpocetine. J Pharm Biomed Anal 1997 Nov;16(3):419-24.

Paleologos M; Cumming RG; et al; *Cohort study of vitamin C intake and cognitive impairment.* University of Sydney, New South Wales, Australia.Am J Epidemiol 1998 Jul 1;148(1):45-50.

Panda S; Kar A Evidence for free radical scavenging activity of Ashwagandha root powder in mice. Indian J Physiol Pharmacol 1997 Oct;41(4):424-6.

Patocka J; Huperzine A--an interesting anticholinesterase compound from the Chinese herbal medicine. Acta Medica (Hradec Kralove) 1998;41(4):155-7.

Prasad MR; Markesbery WR; Regional membrane phospholipid alterations in Alzheimer's disease. Lexington Neurochem Res 1998 Jan;23(1):81-8.

Pudleiner P; Vereczkey L; Study on the absorption of vinpocetine and apovincaminic acid. Chemical Works of Gedeon Richter Ltd, Budapest, Hungary. Eur J Drug Metab Pharmacokinet 1993 Oct-Dec;18(4):317-21.

Ramassamy, C, et al, The Ginkgo biloba extract, Egb761, increases synaptosomal uptake of 5-hydroxytryptamine: in vitro and ex-vico studies, J Pharm Pharmacol 44(11)943-945, 1992.

Riviere S; Birlouez-Aragon I; Nourhashemi F; Vellas B; *Low plasma vitamin C in Alzheimer patients despite an adequate diet.* Int J Geriatr Psychiatry 1998 Nov;13(11):749-54

Secades JJ; Frontera G; CDP-choline: pharmacological and clinical review. Methods Find Exp Clin Pharmacol 1995 Oct;17 Suppl B:2-54.

Shults CW; Haas, RH; Beal, MF; A Possible Role of Coenzyme Q10 in the etiology and treatment of Parkinson's Disease,University of California, San Diego, La Jolla, Neurology Service, VA Health Care System, San Diego, Massachusetts Generai Hospital, Boston.

Singh RB; Treatment.Standard plus Q gel 2caps twice daily showing relief. J of Nutr and Environ Med,UK,1999.

Singh RH; Studies on the Anti-anxiety effect of the Medhya Rasayana Drug (Bacopa Monniera) Department of Kayacikitsa, Institue of Medical Sciences, Banara Hindu University, Varansi-5, India, January 1978.

Sopher BL; Martin GM; Furlong CE; Kavanagh TJ; Neurodegenerative mechanisms in Alzheimer disease. A role for oxidative damage in amyloid beta protein precursor-mediated cell death. Mol Chem Neuropathol 1996 Oct-Dec;29(2-3):153-68

Subhan Z; Hindmarch I; Psychopharmacological effects of vinpocetine in normal healthy volunteers. Eur J Clin Pharmacol 1985;28(5):567-71.

Suemaru S; et al; J Cerebrospinal fluid corticotropin-releasing hormone and ACTH, and peripherally circulating choline-containing phospholipid in senile dementia. Life Sci 1993;53(9):697-706.

Stoll, S., Hartmann, H., et al The potent rree radical scavanger a-Lipoic Acid improved memory in aged mice. Putative relationship to NMDA receptor deficits. Pharmacol. Biochem. Behav (1993) 36:799-805.

Stoll S; Scheuer K; Pohl O; Muller WE Ginkgo biloba extract (EGb 761) independently improves changes in passive avoidance learning and brain membrane fluidity in the aging mouse. Pharmacopsychiatry 1996 Jul;29(4):144-9

Szakall S; Boros I; Balkay L; Emri M; et al; Cerebral effects of a single dose of intravenous vinpocetine in chronic stroke patients: a PET study. Debrecen University Medical School, Hungary. J Neuroimaging 1998 Oct;8(4):197-204.

Tang XC; Huperzine A (shuangyiping): a promising drug for Alzheimer's disease, State Key Lab of Drug Research, Shanghai Institute of Materia Medica, Chinese Academy of Sciences, China. Chung Kuo Yao Li Hsueh Pao 1996 Nov;17(6):481-4.

Tohgi H; Sasaki K; Chiba K; Effect of vinpocetine on oxygen release of hemoglobin and erythrocyte organic polyphosphate concentrations in patients with vascular dementia of the Binswanger type.Arzneimittelforschung 1990 Jun;40(6):640-3.

Yamada K; Tanaka T; Han D; Protective effects of idebenone and alpha-tocopherol on beta-amyloid-(1-42)-induced learning and memory deficits in rats: implication of oxidative stress in beta-amyloid-induced neurotocity in vivo. Eur J Neurosci 1999 Jan;11(1):83-90.

Yazawa, K.; Clinical esperience with DHA in demented patients, International Conference on Highly Unsaturatd Fatty Acids in Nutritio and Desise Prevention, Barcelona, Spain, 1996, November 4-6.

Young SN; The 1989 Borden Award Lecture. Some effects of dietary components (amino acids, carbohydrate, folic acid) on brain serotonin synthesis, mood, and behavior. Can J Physiol Pharmacol 1991 Jul;69(7):893-903.

Zeisel, S. et al.; Dietary Choline: Biochemistry. Physioogy and Pharmacology. Ann. Rev. Nutr. 1981. 1:95-121.

EPILOGUE

After my mother's death, I sent out 50 questionnaires to people who had the opportunity to observe our journey with Moose. I wanted to get a multi-dimensional perspective of Moose's last years. The following are excerpts from those questionnaires.

In response to "Your observations of family with Moose":

Stan P., Ministry at New Life: Your family treated her with respect, dignity, love, great care, patience, understanding, concern, and prayer, walking her to the gates of Heaven. Watching you taught me much. Your love and how you completed your responsibility with love, never complaining, was a joy to observe.

Billy T., Billy's Pizza: *I found love and caring in this family. I was also impressed on how Barry treated Moose and cared for her as he would his own mother.*

Rita C., Social worker at Hospice of the Comforter: *Moose's family was beautiful with her. They were continuously catering to her needs - taking her for rides and eating out. They interacted with her in loving and caring ways. They worked to make her last days on Earth happy ones. She was always clean and comfortable and obviously loved.*

In response to "Interesting, humorous, poignant anecdotes about Moose":

Gwendolyn T., CNA and Personal Care Provider: *When taking Moose for a ride in the car one day, she turned to me and said, "Who do you think you are?" I* realized that we had neglected to ask her if she wanted to go. I found out that this was someone who didn't want to be bossed around or have her feelings taken for granted. Once I informed her of where we were going, and when we should be back, she was fine.

Cheryl W., Personal Care Provider:

1. One day I told Moose her boyfriend was here to see her and she asked, "which one?"

2. I would take Moose around the house with me and I was bent over with my rear end up in the air wiping something off the floor and she said, "Now there's a, there's a, there's a...!" She couldn't find the words, but I knew what she was thinking.

3. Max was at the beginning stages of learning how to play the guitar. He brought it into the living room to proudly show the one or two chords he had learned. After about a minute and a half, Moose said (concerning the guitar), "Sell it, sell it!"

4. While looking at Stan Plesenski's picture, she said, "He's a big, big, big man and I love him!"

Emily M., Personal Care Provider: *Moose was a person that muttered most of the time. Moose would answer with short sentences, such as "Yes," "No," or "I don't want it." In the short time I knew Moose, I found her to be very particular. When I would clean her room or fold laundry, Moose would not mutter. I took this as acceptance of my actions. This led me to believe that Moose was very neat and tidy. When I would insist on trying to feed Moose, she was able to blow out of her mouth whatever she chose not to eat. Chocolate pudding and lemon ice were fine, but tuna salad was NOT.*

ABOUT THE AUTHOR

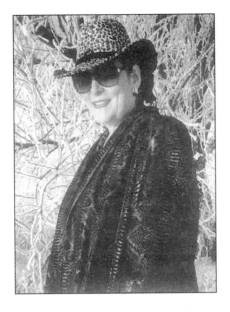

Frances A. (Reinstein) Kraft graduated from Drake University with a degree in secondary education. She taught deaf, emotionally disturbed and retarded students in Chicago, before marrying Barry Kraft.

They have two children, Brandy, 26, married to Dirk Bichsel, and Max, 18. During Barry's Army career, they were stationed in Hawaii, San Francisco, Kansas and Colorado where they spent the last 22 years. There, Fran worked as a beauty consultant for Barbizon Modeling School. In addition, she opened Fran Kraft Reality Co. and was marketing director for an exclusive community.

Recently, the Krafts moved to Pelican Rapids, MN, where they do free Christian counselling and motivational speaking.

Fran currently holds the title of Mrs. Ottertail County and will be competing for Mrs. Minnesota International. She has had articles published in *Bereavement, Hospice* and *Girlfriend Connection* Magazines.

OTHER CONTRIBUTORS

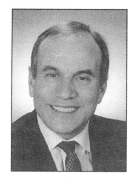

Barry Kraft, D.O., graduated from the College of Osteopathic Medicine and Surgery in Des Moines, Iowa. While serving in the U.S. Army, he took a residency in psychiatry and attained the rank of Colonel, prior to going into private practice.

Before retiring, he was chief of psychiatry at Parkview Medical Center in Pueblo, Co. There, he founded Parkview Family Counselling Center and Parkview Christian Counselling Center and Parkview Inpatient Christian Psychiatry Program. Dr. Kraft was one of the leading authorities on drug and alcohol abuse in Colorado. He also was a national motivational speaker and a frequent guest on Christian radio shows. He has dedicated the last 6 years of his life to serving the Lord full-time.

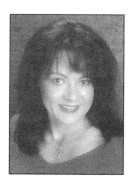

Beth M. Ley, Ph.D., has been a science writer specializing in health and nutrition for over 12 years. She wrote her own undergraduate degree program and graduated in Scientific and Technical Writing from North Dakota State University in 1987 (combination of Zoology and Journalism). Beth has her masters (1997) and doctoral degrees (1999) in Nutrition.

She has written almost 20 different books on health and nutrition, is a frequent guest on radio talk shows and also lectures across the country.

Beth lives in the lake country in Minnesota. She is dedicated to God and to spreading the health message.

Memberships: American Academy of Anti-Aging, New York Academy of Sciences, Oxygen Society.

ORDER THESE GREAT BOOKS
ALSO AVAILABLE FROM BL PUBLICATIONS!

Immune System Control
Colostrum & Lactoferrin

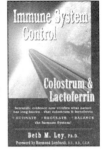

Beth M. Ley, Ph.D. 200 pages, $12.95 ISBN 1-890766-11-9
*Get the indepth and detailed FACTS about colostrum
and lactoferrin! Testimonials and much more! Also features a special product selection guide! Fully refer-
enced/Indexed*

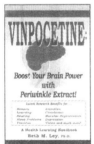

Marvelous Memory Boosters
Beth M. Ley, Ph.D. 2000, 32 pages, $3.95

*Certain nutrients & phytochemicals (Alpha GPC,
Vinpocetine, Huperzine-A, Pregnenolone, Phospholipids,
DHA, Bacopa Monniera, Ginkgo Biloba, etc.) improve
short & long term memory, increase mental acuity & concentration, improve learning abilities & mental stamina,
reduce fatigue, improve sleep, mood, vision & hearing.*

Aspirin Alternatives:
The Top Natural Pain-Relieving Analgesics
Raymond Lombardi, D.C., N.D., C.C.N., 1999, 160 pages, $8.95

*This book discusses analgesics and natural approaches to
pain. Ibuprofen and acetaminophen are used for pain-
relief, but like all drugs, there is a risk of side effects and
interactions. There are a number of natural alternatives
which are equally effective and in many cases may be
preferable because they may help treat the underlying
problem rather than simply treating a symptom.*

Vinpocetine: Boost Your Brain w/ Periwinkle
Extract! Beth M. Ley, Ph.D. 2000, 48 pgs. $4.95

*This herbal extract benefits: Memory, attention and con-
centration, learning, circulation, hearing, insomnia,
depression, tinnitus, vision & more! Vinpocetine increases
circulation in the brain and increases metabolism in the
brain by increasing use of glucose and oxygen. Benefits
both the old and young!*

Coenzyme Q10: All Around
Nutrient for All-Around Health!
Beth M. Ley-Jacobs, Ph.D., 1999, 60 pages, $4.95

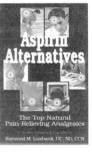

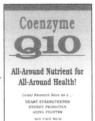

*CoQ10 is found in every living cell. With age, insufficient
levels become more common, putting us at serious risk of
illness and disease. Protect and strengthen the cardiovascular system; benefit blood pressure, immunity, fatigue,
weight problems, Alzheimer's, Parkinson's, Huntington's,
gum-disease and slow aging.*

MSM: On Our Way Back To Health With Sulfur Beth M. Ley, 1998, 40 pages, $3.95

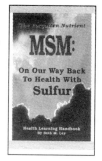

MSM (methyl sulfonyl methane), is a rich source of organic sulfur, important for connective tissue regeneration. Beneficial for arthritis and other joint problems, allergies, asthma, skin problems, TMJ, periodontal conditions, pain relief, and much more! Includes important "How to use" directions.

How to Fight Osteoporosis & Win: The Miracle of MCHC
Beth M. Ley, 80 pgs. $6.95

Find out if you are at risk for osteoporosis and what to do to prevent and reverse it. Get the truth about bone loss, calcium, supplements, foods, MCHC & much more! Find out what supplements can help you most!

DHA: The Magnificent Marine Oil
Beth M. Ley-Jacobs, Ph.D., 1999, 120 pages, $6.95

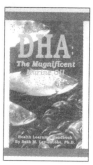

Individuals commonly lack this essential Omega-3 fatty acid so important to the brain, vision, and immune system and much more. Memory, depression, ADD, addiction disorders (especially alcoholism), inflammatory disorders, skin problems, schizophrenia, elevated blood lipids, etc., benefit from DHA.

Colostrum: Nature's Gift to The Immune System-2nd Edition - Revised and Updated
Beth M. Ley, Ph.D. 80 pages, $5.95

Colostrum, "first milk," is rich in immuno-factors such as antibodies, growth factors, lactoferrin, etc., which can boost & support the immune system of everyone!

Phyto-Nutrients: Medicinal Nutrients Found in Foods, Beth M. Ley, 40 pgs. $3.95

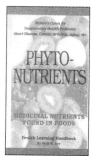

Learn about special components in our foods which protect our health by fighting off disease & aging! Learn about onions, garlic, flax, bilberry, green tea, red wine, rosemary, cruciferous vegetables, cayenne pepper, ginger, soybeans, avocados, beets, cranberries, sweet potatoes, amaranth, etc.

Nature's Road to Recovery: Nutritional Supplements for The Alcoholic & Chemical-Dependent Beth M. Ley-Jacobs, Ph.D., 1999, 72 pages, $5.95

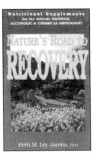

Recovery involves much more than abstinence. Cravings, depression, memory loss, liver problems, vascular problems, sexual problems, sleep problems, nutritional deficiencies and common health problems which can benefit from 5-HTP, DHA, phospholipids, St. John's Wort, antioxidants, etc.

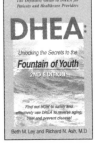

Health Benefits of Probiotics
Dr. S.K. Dash & Dr. Allen Spreen 2000, 56 pages, $4.95

Probiotics aid in the maintenance of the healthy balance of intestinal flora. They improve digestion, cholesterol levels, immunity; Correct digestive disorders, ulcers, inflammatory bowel diseases, lactose intolerance, yeast infections; Help prevent colon cancer; Reduce side effects of antibiotics & more!

DHEA: Unlocking the Secrets to the Fountain of Youth - 2nd Ed. Richard Ash, M.D., & Beth M. Ley, 320 pgs. $14.95

Find how to use the famed "anti-aging hormone," DHEA, safely, without side effects, to reverse aging & treat & prevent disease.

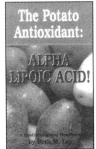

The Potato Antioxidant: Alpha Lipoic Acid
Beth M. Ley, 96 pgs. $6.95

A must read for those with diabetes, cataracts, macular degeneration, HIV & those concerned about aging! Lipoic acid is both fat and water soluble so provides superior antioxidant protection. It is proven to help circulatory disorders such as peripheral neuropathy, improve glucose utilization, protect the eyes against degenerative conditions and more.

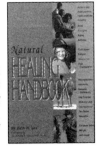

Natural Healing Handbook
Beth M. Ley, 320 pgs. $14.95

Excellent, easy -to-use reference book with natural health care remedies for all your healthcare concerns. A book you will use over & over again!

Look for these titles from BL PUBLICATIONS in your local health food or book stores or

FADING

A great gift to share with friends and loved ones!

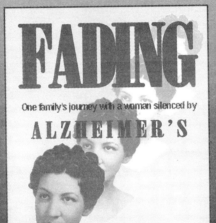

$12.95
plus $2.00 shipping

To order additional copies of **FADING**,
please send check or money order to:
Frances Kraft. P.O. Box 395,
Pelican Rapids, MN 56572-0395.

For speaking engagements, please call 218-863-2469